A WOMAN'S GUIDE TO STAYING HEALTHY THROUGH HER 30s

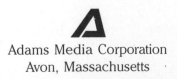

Theresa Francis-Cheung

Adams Media Corporation
Avon, Massachusetts

Published by
Adams Media Corporation
57 Littlefield Street, Avon, MA 02322
www.adamsmedia.com

ISBN: 1-58062-562-2

Printed in Canada.

J I H G F E D C B A

Library of Congress Cataloging-in-Publication Data
Francis-Cheung, Theresa.
A woman's guide to staying healthy through her 30s /
by Theresa Francis-Cheung.
p.   cm.
Includes index.
ISBN 1-58062-562-2
1. Women–Health and hygiene. I. Title.
RA778 .F77   2001
613'.04244–dc21   2001046344

This publication is designed to provide accurate and authoritative information
with regard to the subject matter covered. It is sold with the understanding
that the publisher is not engaged in rendering legal, accounting, or other
professional advice. If legal advice or other expert assistance is required, the
services of a competent professional person should be sought.
—From a *Declaration of Principles* jointly adopted by a Committee of the
American Bar Association and a Committee of Publishers and Associations

Illustration by Joan Farber/Vicki Prentice Associates Inc.

This book is available at quantity discounts for bulk purchases.
For information, call 1-800-872-5627.

Contents

Part One: The Decade of Transition

Part Two: Age-Related Changes

Part Three: Healthy Living in the 30s

Part Four: Everyone Ages

List of Illustrations

Acknowledgments

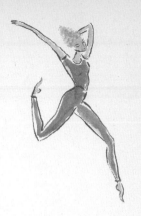

Special thanks to all the women who spent time talking to me about their 30s; their stories gave this project meaning. Their insights are in this book, with names changed to protect identity. I would also like to thank the health professionals and beauty experts who helped provide information about health and aging in the 30s. In particular, I am grateful to Dr. James Douglas, reproductive endocrinologist, and Dr. Arlene Jacobs, gynecologist, from the Plano Medical Center in Texas.

I am truly grateful to all the staff at Adams Media, in particular my editor, Cheryl Kimball, for her encouragement, advice, and inspiration. I am also indebted to Dr. Priscilla Stuckey for her insight and fine developmental editing.

Thanks also to my brother Terry and his partner Robin, and for the support of family and friends. Finally, special gratitude to my husband Ray and son Robert for their patience, support, enthusiasm, and love while I went into exile to do this project.

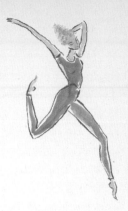

Introduction

"After thirty the body has a mind of its own," said Bette Midler, and many of us in our 30s have learned that she was right. It is one of nature's cruel surprises that just when you leave adolescent insecurities about your body behind, it starts getting unpredictable. You get cellulite and tiny wrinkles. You start to look older.

If you are anxious enough—and most of us are when it comes to our bodies—it will not take you long to find evidence that the first bloom of youth has passed. You may even have a list of complaints similar to those your mom and grandmother might talk about: aches and pains, crow's-feet around the eyes, age spots, extra weight in the hips, varicose veins, and forgetfulness.

The 30s are a decade of transition—physically, mentally, and emotionally. When you look in a mirror you don't see a girl anymore, you see a woman looking back at you. In a culture obsessed with youth and images of pre-30s beauty, the first encounter with adulthood can cause feelings of anxiety. But your concerns are unlikely to be taken seriously. The late 20s to the early 40s are the most neglected and underreported period in a woman's life.

Despite growing interest in the thirtysomething lifestyle generated by books like *Bridget Jones's Diary* and TV series like *Ally McBeal*, there is little information and advice about health in the 30s. Most of the vast amount of literature on aging is directed to the over-40 age group. The majority of studies about developmental stages in a woman's life focus on adolescence and menopause, with virtually no mention of those of us in our 30s.

When I reached my 30s, I wanted to understand more about my health. What was going on with my body. The changes that were going on in my life. Why I was feeling anxious. With so little advice available, I decided to do my own research. I read every book and article and Web site about aging and developmental stages in a woman's life I could lay my hands on. I consulted medical experts and health and beauty specialists. I talked to dozens of women in their 30s from a variety of backgrounds and with different life circumstances: some were single, some were married, some were mothers, some were childless, some worked, some didn't. It was strangely comforting to find that I was not alone with my doubts and fears. Many of the women I interviewed admitted that becoming 30 had been a crisis point, that getting older had come as an unpleasant shock, that feelings of desperation were not uncommon.

I felt that there was a real need for a book about health in the 30s. The best possible time to defend oneself against the ravages of time is when the subtle, early signs of aging are detected and not later, when they are unmistakable and irreversible. In the words of Maureen West, "What we do in our twenties, thirties, and forties can have a huge impact on how fast we age." In her article "Lifetime of Habits Determine Differences in the Aging Process" West stresses the importance of taking care of yourself earlier if you want to live a long, healthy life (*New York Times* News Service, printed in the *Rochester Post-Bulletin*, November 17, 1997).

Initially, the primary intention of this book was to inform and educate women about bodily changes we experience in the 30s so that firm foundations for successful aging could be laid. But in the process of reviewing my research it became obvious that any discussion about health in the 30s is also a discussion about the big issues we face in the 30s. That talk about getting older cannot be separated from talk about career, relationships, children, and what we really want from our lives. Getting older in the 30s is about so much more than bodily health—it is about intellectual and emotional health, too. How we live and the life choices we make influence how we look and feel.

And so, although primarily about physical health, the book also developed into a more general discussion of women's lives in their 30s. It is about hopes, doubts, and expectations. About lessons learned. About becoming an adult.

Part One focuses on the age 30 transition, including the various rites of passage we face and how the first signs of maturing often prompt a reassessment of the hopes and expectations of the 20s.

Part Two addresses every aspect of health in our 30s, the invisible and visible signs of getting older, like cellulite, wrinkles, weight gain, stretch marks, varicose veins, and thinning hair. Makeup and style is here, as well as information about common concerns that crop up in our 30s: for instance, why you may have more aches and pains, why you might start forgetting things, why you may seem to get more colds, why it can be so much harder to shift weight. The section dealing with hormones focuses on PMS, fertility, irregular periods, hormonal problems, and libido. Lifestyle factors such as eating, drinking, relationships, work, and what you do in your leisure time are also examined. Finally, attention is given to psychological and emotional factors like stress, fear, worry, insights, depression, compulsions, expectations, self-esteem, and body image and how these can impact the aging process.

Chapter 7 aims to take some of the fear and mystery out of perimenopause. It will explain exactly what perimenopause is and what you can expect. Symptoms can appear in the early 30s and you will learn how to deal with them positively through diet, exercise, lifestyle changes, and, if needed, hormonal therapy.

Increasing life span and a healthy balanced lifestyle are the main focus of Parts Three and Four. Case histories of thirtysomething women illustrate various approaches to the maturing process. You will probably recognize a little of yourself in all of them. There will be information and advice to help you create your own battle plan for optimum health, both physical and emotional, in the decade of transition.

Everyone gets older, but vitality, fitness, and true beauty are time-less. When the first signs of age are detected in the 30s, under-standing the physical and emotional changes you are going through and taking better care of yourself are crucial. Now is the time to lay firm foundations for a positive future, to rethink your definition of attractiveness. I hope this book will show you that, although leaving your 20s behind is a reality you can no longer ignore, it is not the beginning of decline. Throughout, the emphasis will be on the 30s being not only the prime of your life but the beginning of the prime of your life—that the best is always yet to come.

PART ONE
THE DECADE OF TRANSITION

"You know you're getting older when you wake up with that morning-after feeling, and you didn't do anything the night before."

—Lois L. Kaufman

•   •   •

"I must be getting older. Regular food and sleep are starting to sound more appealing than regular sex."

—Tracy, age 34

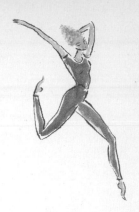

Chapter 1
Age Happens

I am fully aware that the 30s can in no way constitute old age. Talk to any 60-year-old and you will probably get a blank stare, a look of disbelief, or a sigh of exasperation. But I also know that most of us approaching or in our 30s don't know that 30 isn't old.

We are often dumbfounded by the visible changes in our bodies. We aren't sure how to cope with the fears and anxieties we have about leaving childhood behind. And that is why this book has been written. To show you that anxieties about bodily change and fears about being 30 are perfectly natural. You are experiencing a stage in life that just hasn't been discussed that much, that's all. You are not paranoid, pathetic, anxious, or youth obsessed. Your anxieties and fears are a normal part of growing up.

Getting Older

Getting older is a perfectly natural process no woman should fear—it happens to us all. It's impossible to discuss women's health in the 30s without mentioning aging. Your health in your 30s is directly related to the subtle, early signs of the aging process.

And what exactly does aging mean?

The word *aging* is used in two main senses. The first sense is chronological, and tells us that a certain number of years have passed since the umbilical cord was cut. The second sense describes the many changes that have taken place since that moment, some of which are readily available to the eye of the beholder, others perhaps not so easily detected. Or in the words of Nobel Prize winner Linus Pauling, "Aging is the process of growing old and approaching normal death. It is accompanied by a gradual deterioration in the biochemical and physiological functions." Biological aging could then be described as the visible and invisible changes in the cells and tissues that increase the risk of death.

We all know about the visible changes. We know that at some time or other getting older may include many of the following: age spots and wrinkles, graying and thinning hair, extra weight and perhaps even flabby muscles and potbellies, loss of about an inch in height, aches and pains, broken bones and hip replacements, weak bladders and incontinence pads, heartburn and indigestion, vulnerability to disease, especially heart disease and cancer, vulnerability to colds and chest infections, forgetting where you parked the car, forgetting what day it is, forgetting the tickets, forgetting where you put your keys, forgetting what you read on this page, reading glasses and hearing aids.

These are changes we can see, but as we age there are also invisible changes taking place at a cellular level. These include a gradually lowering body temperature, the ratio of body fat to muscle doubling, the slow but steady rise of cholesterol and blood pressure, decreased blood flow to the brain and a general decline in fitness levels and stamina. We can't see these changes but we experience them every time we get fatigued or forgetful or notice loss of muscle tone.

There is no escaping the fact that from the moment we are born we are aging. Usually, sometime around our thirtieth birthday, this process becomes exaggerated. In our teens and 20s we may have felt invincible—life over 30 didn't exist, and we thought we would be forever young. But the 30s bring with them not only bodily changes but a keener sense of our own mortality. Days, weeks, years suddenly flash by faster. We realize that we haven't got forever. Aging in the 30s is no longer a concept we discuss but a reality we experience on a day-to-day basis. That's why we don't really need a Nobel Prize winner's explanation or scientific definition of the term aging. We can see it happening to us in the mirror. And from the age of 30 it seems to be happening faster and faster.

Don't be surprised if all this talk about aging makes you feel uneasy. As Betty Friedan rightly points out in her seminal text *The Fountain of Age,* despite reports of advances in our life expectancy and "an increasing obsession with the problem of age" and how to avoid it through various techniques, there is on the whole an absence of positive images of older people (1993, p. 35). Few of us in our 30s can remember a time when older people were respected, venerated even, for their wisdom and experience. We live in a society that is in age denial. Aging has become a problem and a burden.

Social messages make us fully aware of the unpleasant face of aging. Old age is associated with poor health, dependency, and loss of appeal. What is desperately needed in our culture is an understanding of aging that incorporates not just the negative but the positive face of aging. We need to hear more about the refinement, wisdom, maturity, and insight aging brings. We need to see more positive images of the aging process. We need to hear that aging is fun. That aging gives our life meaning. That you can grow old with beauty, health, and vitality. We need to understand that a large part of how we age is really up to us and how we live our lives. We need to hear less about efforts to delay the aging process unnaturally and more about aging naturally with grace and beauty.

And if you are in your 30s you may not know it yet, but you are already on the right track. Simply by reading this book and learning about the physical and emotional changes age brings in the 30s and how to take better care of yourself, you are laying the foundation stones for a healthy approach to aging. And by so doing you are playing your part in encouraging the much needed shift in our society from age denial to age awareness and celebration.

Why Do Some of Us Age Faster Than Others?

Signs of aging in a group of thirtysomething women show an amazing variation. Some look older than others. Some have wrinkles, some don't. Some have cellulite and some don't.

"My friend Lucy is a year older than me and she still looks like a teenager." (Jill, age 30)

"My sister Rickki is 31 but everyone thinks she is my aunt or something. I guess she just looks old for her age." (Sarah, age 28)

Before we briefly examine some of the theories that attempt to explain why we age, why few of us reach our calendar potential, and why some of us look younger than others, so that we can understand where antiaging advice is coming from, we need to be aware of the term "life expectancy."

Scientists estimate that the longest a human living today can hope to live is 120 years. This is the maximum number of years any human has ever lived. 120 years is 1,440 months, 6,240 weeks, 43,800 days, and over a million hours, to be precise. So if you are reading this and you are 30 you have potentially another 90 years to go. But although we have the potential to live to well over a hundred, the reality is that few of us do.

Life expectancy is how long a person can expert to live based on a number of factors, most of which are within our control. If you were born thousands of years ago during the time of the Roman Empire and you were approaching your 30th birthday, you would have been considered elderly. The average age of death was 22. At the time of the American Revolution, average life expectancy was 35. As recent as the turn of the twentieth century, life expectancy was still 50 years. Since then life expectancy has increased by 25 years because of improved standards of living, better health care, and better lifestyle habits. Average life expectancy for a woman today, according to Elizabeth Somer in *Age-Proof Your Body* (1998) is around 76 years.

The big question is, if we have the potential to live to 120 and living conditions have improved so dramatically, why do so few of us make it?

The search for the secret to a longer, healthier life span, why some of us age faster than others, and how to increase life expectancy has intrigued scientists, doctors, and antiaging specialists for centuries. At present, theories of aging that try to understand why some of us age faster than others seem to divide into two groups: those that presume a pre-existing master plan, and those based on random events.

The Master Plan Theories

Chief among the master plan theories is the concept of aging determined by some kind of inner clock within the cell.

In the 1960s it was discovered that cells are not immortal, but preprogrammed to die after dividing a certain number of times. The set number of replications is known as the "Hayflick limit." Human cells have about 55 regenerations. Hayflick proposed that each cell has an internal clock that counts the number of divisions and triggers cell death. According to Hayflick, life span is determined somewhere in the cell. We age according to a master plan.

Exponents of the master plan theory believe that if they could discover where the internal clock is within the cell, it might be possible to stop the clock and modify the aging process. In 1998, huge excitement was generated world wide when it was reported in *Science* magazine that scientists had found a clue to the secret of eternal life. Scientists from the antiaging research company Geron, together with those at the University of Texas Southwestern Medical Center in Dallas, had come up with the theory that the enzyme telomerase could halt the biological aging of cells. Telomerase is that substance that seems to allow cells to carry on dividing rather than going into self-destruct mode. Scientists found that telomerase is present in 85 percent of cancer cells, explaining their indestructibility.

The results of this research have phenomenal implications. It implies that if the telomerase in cancer cells is blocked, it could kill the tumor, and that if telomerase is added to healthy cells, it could stop them from dying off. But researchers are still only cautiously optimistic about the potential. Telomerase is only part of the puzzle of aging and it carries with it a high risk of cancer.

Other theories of aging that are based on genetic design include the neuroendocrine theory. According to this theory, age changes are determined by hormones secreted at a preprogrammed time by the hypothalamus and pituitary gland in the brain, thus making the brain the origin of all age-related change.

The death gene theory offers another explanation. There is a rare disorder called Werner's Syndrome. This disorder speeds up human aging so that even very young adults get osteoporosis, wrinkles, gray hair, and so on. Before they reach the age of 30, Werner patients look like 80-year-olds. Research has shown that there may be a gene responsible for this tragic disorder. Perhaps this is the gene that regulates human aging? Perhaps it signals to the cells to stop their regenerative function? Perhaps in some of us the gene is defective and we age quicker? Would it be possible to do something to this gene to prolong life? Research still has no definitive answers.

The master plan theories tell us that we are stuck with a future we cannot control. Our life timer has been set and this timer is different for each individual—it determines how long our childhood will be, how we will age in our 30s, when we are going into menopause, and when we will die. If this all seems rather depressing and fatalistic, don't despair—even the most brilliant minds in the world have been unable to prove definitively that any one of them is true.

Random Events

Theories of aging based on random events offer explanations that seem more appealing because control isn't completely taken from our hands. They are based in the belief that aging results from accidental events that are random and not purposefully programmed. Such theories might attribute aging to the accumulation of errors in important molecules such as DNA, the results of wear and tear, or the accumulation of waste products. Let's explore a few of them.

The wear and tear theory likens us to machines. Treated well and given the right kind of fuel, the machine will perform well. Abused and left to rust, the machine will not perform optimally. Eventually after years of use, the machine will just break down and stop working.

As we look in the mirror over the years it is easy to believe this idea. Wrinkles, graying hair, and stiff joints may make us feel and look worn out and ready for the scrap yard, but this theory has inconsistencies. First of all, every human being is unique, unlike machines that are produced on a production line. Genetics and lifestyle play a large part in aging. Also, human beings have the ability to regenerate when there is bodily malfunction. Death occurs when the body stops or is unable to repair what is broken. Perhaps the answer lies in what causes the body to stop doing its repair work.

The rate-of-living theory is based on the belief that animals are born with a limited amount of some substance, potential energy or physiological capacity that can be expended at various rates. If it is used up rapidly, aging begins early. If it is consumed slowly, then aging will be slowed. The theory is often referred to as the "live fast, die young" theory.

The starvation theory bases life expectancy on frugality of food intake. Humans have about 80 million calories per pound per lifetime to consume before the system shuts down. So the more frugal your diet, the better chance you have to live to a ripe old age. The trouble with this is that we must eat to live. Also, a diet poor in essential nutrients and vitamins has the opposite effect and increases the risk of premature aging.

The chaos theory suggests that over time the energy that holds us together disintegrates and we succumb to the natural law of decay. This is interesting, but it still does not explain why some of us have more energy than others and live longer.

The waste product theory says that when one of our body's normal waste-removal systems malfunctions, byproducts accumulate and cells are damaged. As we age our body does get less efficient at removing waste and this can cause discomfort. Still, whether there is a direct link between constipation and aging is debatable.

The immune system theory suggests a link between immunity and aging. The body's immune system separates germs from normal cells. Sometimes the immune system malfunctions and starts to attack healthy body tissues, leading to aging. However, whether aging causes or is caused by a poorly functioning immune system is not known. We do know, though, that free radicals, poor diet, and an unhealthy lifestyle can interfere with normal immune function.

According to the cross-linkage theory of aging, cell regeneration stops when there are problems with cell communication. This theory suggests that cells generate defective messengers that tell the cells to produce defective or cross-linked proteins and enzymes. The migrant molecules accumulate and eventually interfere with normal cell function or cause cell death. They attach themselves to our joints and muscles causing that familiar stiffness we all feel from time to time, especially first thing in the morning. The longer we live, the more webs we have. Eventually the whole system stiffens and we die.

This is an interesting theory. The wonderful flexibility of a baby compared to the stiffness of a corpse makes it even more credible. However, not all of us get stiffer and stiffer as we get older, so there must be something that can help us fight this stiffness. Another question is what causes these defective molecules. No one really knows for sure, but many researchers believe that compounds called free radicals are the culprits.

In several of the theories mentioned previously, free radicals have been suggested as contributory factors in aging. The free radical theory does offer an attractive explanation to the aging process. It also shows us a way to try and slow this process down.

So what are free radicals? Free radicals are highly reactive compounds that can attack and damage the genetic code and membranes of cells and prevent energy production. Have you ever looked at what oxygen does to metal? Free radicals make it rust. What about that apple you took a bite out of? Free radicals make it go brown. What about that milk you forgot to put in the fridge? Free radicals make it go sour. What about the wrinkles on your face? Free radicals and oxygen are the culprits.

According to this theory, the body can be damaged by oxygen and free radicals found in air pollution and normal metabolic processes. Free radicals damage the cell membranes and the cell's power house, called the mitochondria. How do free radicals enter our body? We breathe them in; we produce them when we eat a meal, every time our heart beats, every time we think. Free radicals are the byproducts of living. There is nothing we can do about them. They are a part of life.

It is thought that our bodies suffer around ten thousand free radical hits a day. Over the years the cells become damaged or abnormal. The immune system weakens and we are more susceptible to colds and illness. Damage caused by free radicals seems to escalate over the age of 30. Fortunately, the body has defense mechanisms in the form of vitamins, minerals, enzymes, and other compounds known as the antioxidant system. Antioxidants can clear away free radicals.

Minimizing lifestyle habits that promote free radicals is another form of defense. A healthy lifestyle minimizes the risk of free radical damage. Through breathing, eating, and drinking, the body's defense system can normally disarm free radicals. However, we often are the agents of further free radical damage. Every time we eat too much fat, or smoke, or breathe in polluted air, or stock up on junk food, or drink too much alcohol, we open the doors to free radical attacks that can age us. Later in the book there is more information about antioxidants and lifestyle changes that minimize the chance of free radical damage.

The abuse theory in many ways complements the free radical

theory. Both theories encourage us to treat our bodies well to slow down the aging process. Research has shown that those who live the longest eat a sensible low-fat, high-fiber diet; exercise regularly; avoid alcohol, tobacco, and drugs; watch their weight; have a positive attitude; visit a doctor when needed; have a positive approach to stress; are educated; have the support of friends and family; and have enough money to feel independent. Those who live the shortest, on the other hand, don't take care of themselves and indulge in unhealthy pursuits like smoking.

This sounds attractive, but we all know or have heard of some feisty lady who lived to 100 and smoked and drank too much all her life. What was her secret?

Some experts believe that the underlying molecular process of aging is due to increasing hormonal miscommunication. Hormones direct and coordinate every bodily function. A hormone is a biochemical messenger that communicates information with incredible speed. If anything goes wrong with that hormonal communication system because of stress, disease, poor diet, and so on, you age faster than you should. As we age, hormonal miscommunication increases and systems controlled by hormonal messengers malfunction. The most notable effects are excess free radicals, excess blood glucose, excess cortisol, and excess insulin, all of which increase the formation of aging.

The love and survival theory is based on a simple but powerful theory. Our survival depends on the healing power of love, intimacy, and relationships—as communities, as a country, as a culture, perhaps even as a species. For the past 20 years, research spearheaded by Dr. Dean Ornish has demonstrated that love and intimacy and the emotional and spiritual transformation that often results are the most powerful and meaningful intervention in life expectancy. These are factors that are largely ignored by the medical profession, which tends to focus primarily on the physical and mechanistic: drugs and surgery, genes and germs, microbes and molecules. Ornish argues that love and intimacy are the root of what makes us sick and well, what causes sadness and what brings happiness, what makes us suffer and what leads to healing, and ultimately what can prolong our life.

Certainly lack of meaningful relationships and loneliness can take away the will to live, but the love and survival theory will probably always remain just that: a theory.

And last, but by no means least, the quantum alternative to aging offers a fascinating answer to the question of aging. This theory postulates that the secret to conquering the universal mystery of aging lies not in our bodies but in our consciousness. Arguing that the body is not an object but a process whose limits are not known, exponents of this theory, notably Dr. Deepak Chopra, suggest that the effects of aging are largely preventable by our conscious and unconscious thoughts, emotions, and conditioned attitudes.

The biochemistry of the body is a product of awareness, beliefs, thoughts, and emotions, and creates the chemical reactions that uphold life in every cell. An aging cell is the end product of awareness that has forgotten how to remain new. Basically, when we believe ourselves to be old, we are.

So Why Do We Age?

Now that we have looked at some of the many explanations offered for why we age, what can we conclude? Why do some of us in our 30s notice the early signs of aging before others? The truth is that we still do not know. There will always be exceptions to disprove each theory because no two women will age in the same way. We are all unique. In the future we may well find the answer to one of life's greatest mysteries, but for now perhaps the easiest explanation is to suggest that every theory has something to recommend it. We can learn something from all of them; aging has many causes.

At the annual meeting of the American Association for the Advancement of Science in 1992, Professor Michael Rose of the

University of California announced that in time increasing the life expectancy and human life span will not be inconceivable. "Aging used to be mysterious," he declared, "and now it isn't." Maybe one day we will understand exactly why and how we age. But that is in the future. For now research shows that even though every woman is unique, there are things all of us can do to increase life expectancy and feel years younger.

Rather than accepting that we are stuck with a life span that is out of our control, or that aging follows a certain preprogrammed pattern, we are offered an exciting alternative. Research has shown that poor diet, too much sun, lack of exercise, stressful situations, and emotions that cause anger, fear, and frustration can speed up the aging process. You can delay aging and combat the wear and tear factor by stalling the action of free radicals. Scientists and doctors believe that the sooner we start making antiaging lifestyle changes, the greater our chances of longevity.

Increasingly scientists are coming to the conclusion that the way we live our lives is the determining factor for life expectancy. "Much of what we consider getting older is a reflection of what we think and how we live" (Somer, p. 7). How we live our lives: what we eat, what we drink, how much we exercise, how we react to stress, what we think, and what we feel are all decisive factors. And all these factors are under our control. We are being encouraged to take responsibility for how we age, so that even though we may age chronologically, we don't have to look and feel old.

Now that we've looked at some of the many explanations about age-related change, let's take a brief look at how we can expect to change over the years.

Mirror, Mirror on the Wall

Millions of us keep track of the aging process with our mirrors. Before we move on to examine in detail age-related changes in the 30s, let's consider all the decades of a woman's life, what we typically can and can't see as we watch our face and body change.

Remember, though, these images are of what *might be* but not necessarily what *will be*. They represent what generally happens, not what always happens. Every woman is unique. This book in no way intends to make you obsess about bodily changes. The stress of this will age you even quicker! The intention is that you are forewarned and hopefully forearmed against visible and invisible signs of change.

The 20s: The Decade of Experimentation

She looks young. She is at her so-called "peak" and experiencing maximum physical, sexual, and reproductive capacity. As she approaches 30, though, the first signs of aging begin to appear. There is loss of muscle tone. Her hearing in the high register begins to fade. The rate at which her body burns calories begins to slow down. From now on her metabolic rate will drop by 2 percent a decade.

Remember the 20s. You may have had puppy fat which gave your face less interesting definition than it has now, but you could live on Diet Coke, Mars bars, and junk food and not put on too much weight. You could forget to take your make up off and not need moisturizer. You could stay up all night and not look terrible the next day. You could see a wrinkle-free reflection in the mirror.

It is a tragedy that in the decade when we really don't have to worry too much about our appearance, the great majority of us hate the way we look! Many studies show that poor body image, perhaps caused by unresolved childhood conflicts, is possibly the greatest stress factor in the 20s. It can make young women look far older than they really are. Many women I talked to in their 30s who suffered from body image anxiety in their teens and 20s felt that obsessive thoughts, compulsions, and insecurity destroyed the fun and spontaneity of the 20s.

The 20s are the decade of experimentation. Smoking, drugs, junk food, and alcohol probably didn't bother you. You may even have been convinced that coffee and smoking kept your weight down. You felt young and indestructible and couldn't conceive of a time when you wouldn't want your ears pierced five times or your hair bleached. However, it is worth establishing good habits in the 20s. Smoking, tanning, a poor diet, and too little or too much exercise will prematurely age you. Many women in their 20s are not as fit as they were in their teens, and lack of a regular exercise routine could set them up for weight problems later. Others exercise too much and put themselves at risk of osteoporosis and menstrual problems.

The 30s: The Decade of Transition

Age spots might begin to appear, along with crow's-feet around her eyes and laugh lines around her mouth. Her skin won't give her as much protection from the sun's rays. In her mid-30s there is a gradual loss of bone strength. There is also a gradual loss of cardiovascular fitness, which can drop as much as 40 percent by the age of 65. She may also notice a slight weight gain. But she has lost that baby-faced roundness of her 20s. Her features may be more sharply defined. She may also have the emotional maturity she perhaps lacked in her 20s to really enjoy her sexuality.

The 30s is the decade when you are fully adult and have left your childhood behind. Stresses that can be aging in this decade have been outlined previously. Principal among these are the need to establish your independence, the ticking of the biological clock, conflict between what you want out of life and what others expect from you, and the brutal realization that your looks are not going to be the same forever.

This is the decade when you will first recognize the visible signs of the biological process of aging, when you realize that age happens, even to you.

The 40s: The Decade to Reassess

Skin becomes drier, thinner, and is probably not wrinkle-free, especially if she enjoys getting a tan. There could be dark lines or bags under her eyes. She could need reading glasses now, as the lenses in her eyes have been stiffening since her early 40s, making it hard for her to read small print. She could start seeing more and more gray hair. Perimenopausal symptoms could set in. But intellectually and emotionally, she is more focused than ever.

A woman in her 40s often wonders if she has achieved her goals. She may feel the need to reassess every aspect of her life. This can be a stressful and critical decade. It is the beginning of the second half of life, and a great time to create change if there is frustration and lack of fulfillment.

Perimenopausal symptoms can start as early as 35, but they usually start in the 40s. There might be short-term memory loss. Libido may decrease but more often than not women in their 40s find that it increases. Many women say that the 40s are their sexual peak. Unfortunately men of the same age may not be quite so enthusiastic, as male testosterone levels decline in the 40s. This can cause relationship problems.

Changing weight can be aging in this decade. Women in their 40s start to look older when they lose weight, because it is more difficult to maintain muscle mass as arm muscles, buttocks, and breasts start to sag. Weight tends to spread around the middle. Hair tends to get thinner and the odd gray hair will probably appear. Shampooing every day and massaging the head exercises the scalp and encourages healthier hair growth. Few women in their 40s will be without wrinkles. Keeping face and hands clean and moisturized and using foundations that protect from the sun will help.

Changes in appearance can make a woman wonder if she is still attractive. Keeping active mentally and physically is vital for successful aging. Eating a diet rich in antioxidants, keeping away from the sun, and being alert to bodily change is also important. If a woman can navigate her way through all the challenges of the 40s she can emerge stronger, more energetic, and more vital than ever before.

The 50s: The Decade of Freedom

Ovaries stop producing estrogen and progesterone around the age of 50. Fifty-one is the average age of menopause. Declining hormone levels during and after menopause accelerate bone loss, reduce vaginal lubrication, and raise cholesterol levels, increasing the risk of heart attack and osteoporosis. Skin tone will be more irregular, and it could loosen and sag in certain places like the cheeks and neck. But with her reproductive life behind her she can enjoy a newfound sense of freedom and independence.

Stresses that can age in this decade include the empty nest syndrome when children leave home. It is still possible to have a child, but coming to terms with the loss of reproductive function can be a major readjustment.

This is the decade when many women enjoy a newfound sense of freedom and independence. As far as work is concerned, this can be the power decade for women when positions of authority are often reached. A sense of adventure, a sense of humor, ensuring that there is as much laughter and love in her life as possible, and avoiding aging emotions like fear, anger, and frustration is how she can stay looking and feeling young.

The 60s: The Decade of Resilience

She now begins to grow ever so slightly shorter. Over the next 20 years she'll lose about half an inch in height. She will look less toned as muscle continues to be replaced by fat. She may find that she's a size or two smaller than before and loses some weight, since muscle weighs more than fat. Her skin will look tougher and there may be marks and splotches. She's also more likely to pick up viruses as her immune system isn't as strong as it used to be. But if she has taken care of her body and her mind, age can bring wisdom and resilience.

This is the decade when being about 10 pounds heavier might

actually make a woman look younger. A plumper face can look less wrinkled. Keeping body-conscious and getting regular exercise to counteract bone loss is important.

A sixtysomething woman may find that work opportunities decline. She could be more vulnerable to illnesses and infection. It is vital in this decade that she keeps positive, busy, and exercises both body and mind. If she challenges herself, stays current, and doesn't live in the past, age can bring beauty, wisdom, and resilience.

The 70s and Beyond: The Decades to Celebrate

Reduced muscle tone means that she might have problems with incontinence. Her digestion won't be as efficient either. She needs a lot of light to see clearly and a lot more time to do simple daily tasks. However, if she has kept her mind active she can be as lively and mentally focused as ever. These are the decades when she can look back at her past with understanding. The wisdom gained from every experience will help her enjoy and celebrate her life.

One of the biggest dangers here is boredom. A seventysomething woman should try not to rely on others to do everything for her. She needs to stay active mentally and physically, have goals and interests, and keep learning and growing. Loss of independence due to ill health is a fear and a worry. But if she has taken good care of her body and her mind and seeks fulfillment, pleasure, and happiness from all that she does she will have a timeless vitality that keeps her looking and feeling young. She will have aged but she won't seem old.

It's Not Too Late

Don't get despondent if you spent most of your teens and 20s dieting, feeling stressed, and getting a tan. Hopefully you will have seen that it's never too late to improve your health and fitness. The mirror has shown us that each decade has its joys, challenges, and sorrows. Looking older, when you first begin to notice it in your 30s, is not something to be feared, but a perfectly natural process that brings with it gains as well as losses. Remember, leaving your youth behind doesn't have to be about stagnation and failing health.

Aging Yesterday and Today

Age happens, but how it happens and whether or not we look older than we should is, to a certain extent, up to us.

We don't have to age in the same way that our mothers and grandmothers did. "Aging today is not like it was for our mothers," write the editors of *Prevention* magazine in *Age Erasers for Women: Actions You Can Take Right Now to Look Younger and Feel Great* (1994, p. 3). Our moms or grandmoms may have typically put on a good ten pounds at age 30, had dry skin at 35, gum disease at 40, stiff joints and backs at 45, high cholesterol at 50, heart disease at 55, and forgetfulness and osteoporosis at 60. But we don't have to age like that.

Aging today is not like it was for past generations of women because we know that we can avoid weight gain, heart disease, osteoporosis, and high cholesterol through diet and exercise. Wrinkles can be prevented if we use sunscreen. Age spots and dry or oily skin are largely preventable through diet. Keeping our minds active can keep our brains young. We know that extra weight, aches and pains, wrinkles, memory loss, and so on can make us look old, but that the real cause of aging is in the way we live our lives. "The real age-maker is not physical. . . . Aging is for the most part what we do to ourselves" (p. 4).

A great deal of the aging process is up to you. Even though it's impossible to stop age-related change, you can at least slow it down. By making certain lifestyle changes you don't have to look older than you are. In the words of Mary Spillane and Victoria McKee in *Ultra Age: Every Woman's Guide to Facing the Future*, "We are all guilty in some way of accelerating the aging process," but there is a difference between the normal wear and tear of everyday living and indulging in activities which are damaging to our bodies (1999, p. 83).

Put simply, getting old is eating a high-calorie, high-fat diet, smoking and drinking too much, lying in the sun, watching too much television, and avoiding mental and physical challenge. Aging is about apathy. Aging is giving up on life and giving up on yourself.

And aging doesn't start when most of us think it starts. You don't suddenly wake up one morning in your sixties and look old. Technically, you are aging from birth, even though you won't notice visible changes 'till you hit your 30s, which seems to be the decade when looking older than your years isn't cool anymore.

It's never too early to start thinking about how well you will age. The sooner you start taking care of your body and mind, the more likely it is that you will hold on to your youthful health. And making lifestyle changes in the 30s is, according to many antiaging experts, the optimum time. Young enough to start a new regime of health care and hopefully old enough to have learned from your mistakes, you can prepare a bright and exciting agenda to maintain youthful vitality.

Research is also proving that it's not only bodily health but how we think, how we feel, and how much stress there is in our lives that matter. There are psychological and emotional aging factors to take into account. Signs of bodily decline are only a part of the story of aging in the 30s. A healthy lifestyle is not just about physical health. Emotional, intellectual, and spiritual satisfaction are equally important. Before discussing the physical signs of aging, I will focus on typical psychological and emotional issues of the 30s which, depending on how we cope with them, can age or rejuvenate us.

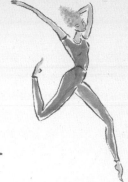

Chapter 2
The Turbulent 30s

The expectation is that by the age of 30 you have finally grown up. Your life is nicely in order and there is a maturity in everything you do. The reality is that many of us find the prospect of 30 terrifying.

"I woke up on the morning of my thirtieth birthday with a feeling of dread. Wasn't I supposed to be married and responsible by now?" (Linda, age 30)

"I just couldn't imagine myself being thirty when I was a teenager. It seemed really old." (Rebecca, age 31)

A vague sense of panic or impending doom often accompanies the late 20s. Perhaps you never imagined life beyond the teens and the 20s. You have no images of yourself getting older. You have no idea what life has in store for you and how you will cope with it. You grew up thinking that you should "never trust anyone over thirty." What happens now that you yourself are actually entering your 30s?

Or perhaps you had hoped to be "somebody" by the age of 30. Independent, successful, and happy. Instead you feel that you haven't found your path in life. Nancy, age 38, remembers how she would spend hours talking with her school friends. "We decided that when we were thirty we would still be friends. Our kids would play together and we would drink lemonade in the garden. Life would be without stress. We would be free. I had no idea then how hard growing up is. How tough life can be."

Few women approaching their thirtieth birthday will be without

23

anxiety. Friends and family constantly remind us that 30 is just around the corner. The loss of youth becomes the butt of everyone's jokes. The birthday party seems more like a funeral than a celebration. Birthday card greetings try to inject humor into the situation, but all they do is trivialize it. Here's a snapshot of some of the cards I got when I hit the big 3-0!

- Happy 30th Birthday! Inside this card is a list of all the good points about being 30. (the card is blank inside)
- 30th Birthday Wishes
  You are charming, sweet, and bold,
  daring, dashing, remarkable, and old.
- Congratulations for getting this far. There is something I must tell you. You are now . . . officially old.

On a good day the cynicism may make us smile but on bad days it may have the opposite effect. It trivializes and makes light of what is an important turning point. And it's no good trying to look for sympathy. Apart from friends the same age who may empathize, everyone else will save their concern for those approaching mid-life. And quite rightly so. Alongside a 70-year-old you may even feel faintly ridiculous for feeling anxious. But, despite all attempts at rational thinking, when paranoia strikes it seems unfair that few people will take seriously your concern that 30 is a crisis point. Your thirtieth birthday party can be a lonely one, regardless of how many guests you invite.

Big Issues in the 30s

When I talked to thirtysomething women about their lives, a sense of restlessness and crisis was obvious. I also noticed that they tended to talk about their lives in categories or themes. There was their love life, their sex life, their social life, their work, their bodies, and how they felt about themselves. Sometimes one or two aspects of their life seemed to be going well, but they felt that the others weren't.

"Now I'm in my thirties, it's so hard to be successful in every area of my life," says Helen, age 33. "At the beginning of the year I had a great social life. Lots of friends and parties and things to do. Work was going well but I missed having a special relationship. The year before last I had a boyfriend but I felt miserable. Now I have a boyfriend again and I feel happier but I'm putting on weight and I've missed out on a promotion at work."

As we examine these big themes in more detail, it is important to point out that what follows is simply a cross section of views and insights from thirtysomething women, some of which you may relate to and some of which you may not. Admittedly, the 30s are a time of transition, and there may be similarities in the issues and crises we face, but how each individual experiences them will be unique to her. I haven't cross-sectioned each reference here because the ways in which to cope with the emotional and psychological challenges of the 30s will be dealt with in more detail later.

Love Life

By the time we are in our 30s, most of us have had time alone between romantic relationships. Having this time alone can be strengthening in many ways.

Some women find that they actually prefer being alone. Sophia, 34, admits that although she has not ruled marriage out she can't see it happening to her. Other women find that being alone builds their self-esteem. "I used to envy a friend of mine who married when she was eighteen," says Nina, age 32. "She seemed so safe and happy with a husband, a house, and two kids. Recently she confided in me that she had always envied me. Everything had always been done for her. She didn't know if she had it in her to make it alone like I had. What she said made me realize how much I had achieved and how proud I should be of myself."

Feeling capable of handling things yourself is something that may suddenly become very important in the 30s. It's all part of the struggle for adulthood. In your 30s it's embarrassing to get handouts from parents. Getting things the easy way just doesn't seem right. There is nothing more rewarding than working for something yourself. But just when you may be enjoying this newfound sense of independence, suddenly the pressure is on you to find the right person and become a couple.

Women of our generation were encouraged to establish their careers before marriage. As a result, the number of single women in their 30s is rising. *Bridget Jones's Diary* (1998) has immortalized the supposed trials and tribulations of a single woman in her 30s.

Bridget Jones's Diary was an instant success because it captured so well the classic thirtysomething angst about food, drinking, cigarettes, weight, men, career, and friendship. Bridget begins her new year in a single bed in her parents' house. "It is too humiliating at my age," she confides. "How does a woman get to your age without being married?" she is asked as she is introduced at a Christmas party. Bridget's insecurity about her looks, her life, and her capacity to attract men and sustain a relationship with a responsible adult make compulsive and hilarious reading, because, however confident we may think we are, we have all been there.

The prejudice against single women in their 30s is no myth. The image of the frustrated, neurotic spinster is deep-seated. Many of the single women I talked to said that they were fed up with being pitied and being set up for blind dates as if their friends were uncomfortable with the idea of a single female in her 30s. Margaret, who was 36 when she got married, describes how relieved family and friends seemed to be. "I could have got married when I was younger. But I take marriage seriously. I wanted to wait for the right person. I did think when I was a girl that I'd be married by the time I reached thirty but it just didn't happen."

Many single women admitted that being a thirtysomething single woman wasn't easy, that they were starting to lower their standards.

"By this stage in life most of the decent men have been snapped up," says Sarah, age 34. The increasing earning power and economic status of women who are in their 30s and single has led to many being prepared to embrace men they might previously have regarded as inferior—intellectually, economically, and socially.

Cultural messages bombard us about marriage and happiness and spinsterhood, loneliness, bitterness, and neurosis, despite the fact that married women have a much higher rate of depression than single women and feminists criticize it is as an inherently male institution. No matter how many happy unattached women there are, the rest of society seems to insist that being 30-plus and single equals being sad. This feeling is represented in the recent surge in thirtysomething novels about life in the single lane, of which *Bridget Jones* is the best example. The heroines are either too fat, too lonely, or both, and their lives are full of disastrous experiences with men. The message is usually the same: life without a man is not worth living.

It's no surprise that given this pressure, some women start to create imaginary boyfriends or fantasize about relationships that have no chance of being realized. "I had this one date with a gorgeous guy," says Amanda, age 36. "He's gone abroad now for a new job but he's the man of my dreams. I know that we are meant to be together."

Whatever your views on relationships and marriage and however well you cope with being single, one thing is clear: It is not a passport to instant fulfillment and happiness. It is not always the happily ever after. A partner, male or female, is not going to make everything right. "It was a big shock to me," says Sandy, age 31, "when after a whirlwind romance and an exciting wedding I still couldn't come to terms with my depression. I still felt restless. I was still searching for meaning."

You may prefer the single life. Kate, age 33, admits that she feels a pang of regret when she is once again the bridesmaid and not the bride, and she is sick of being looked at as if she is some kind of freak because her biological clock is ticking, but this is not reason enough for her to give up the single lifestyle she loves. "No matter how often my grandmother wrings her hands in despair and tells me I'm not getting any younger, I don't actually want a committed relationship." If, however, you are less committed to the single life than Kate and more relationship-minded, there is no need to go into a panic in your 30s.

Single thirtysomething women are the fastest growing social group. Being alone in your 30s is not really a big deal anymore. Women are getting educated. Establishing careers. Living their lives. There is no harm in waiting. You can take your time. There are other things in life besides marriage, and studies show that marriages made later in life tend to last longer than marriages made earlier. "We've been socialized to think that 30 is the drop-dead cutoff for institutions like marriage" writes Julie Tilsner in *29 and Counting* (1998, p. 116). But 30 is still quite a young age to have the wisdom and self-knowledge to recognize the partner of your dreams.

Thankfully, attitudes are changing as single women begin to talk openly about their lives and why they chose to remain single. Most of us have a clearer understanding of what we do and don't want as far as our love life is concerned. Our past experiences will have taught us, according to Lauren Dockett and Kristin Beck in *Facing 30: Women Talk about Constructing a Real Life and Other Scary Rites of Passage,* that perhaps "some of us do know something about our hearts" even if we don't really understand love itself (1998, p. 80).

Some of us in our 30s may have lost our youthful optimism about love and commitment. Andrea, age 31, says that when she was young she dreamed of the fairy tale happily ever after. "But now I've accepted being alone. If you become the sum total of your past, then mine has made me deeply cautious of men. In my thirties, I wonder if I will ever find a soulmate."

Disappointments may make us have doubts about the future. We don't think about love and marriage the way our parents did. We wonder how much we were to blame for the failure of relationships in the past. Part of us may long for the happily ever after, but most of us are coming to terms with the idea that falling in love may not always be forever. We may feel cynical about our future. Sarah, age 33, is "pessimistic about marriage. I've seen too many of my friends divorce." On the other hand, Victoria, age 39, has married and divorced twice. She doesn't regret any of her relationships. "They were right at the time. At the moment there is no one special. I'd like there to be but I don't mind being alone either."

We have all read about the high divorce statistics—at least one in five marriages fail. Perhaps our own parents' marriage failed. The fairy tale marriage of Charles and Diana failed. The institution of marriage and the notion of commitment have received a lot of knocks. For Elizabeth, age 30, the idea of marriage doesn't appeal at all. "At the moment I really don't want to get married. There are lots of people I want to be intimate with. I couldn't just focus on the one person."

Difficulties with your love life and frustration that you may never find the partner of your dreams can be psychologically stressful and aging. It can be very difficult to find the happy medium. We want to do our own thing, but we also want to share. We want to feel free, but we also want commitment. "I really loved Judy," says Rosie, age 34. "I just wasn't ready to say that this was the relationship. I miss her now she has gone, but I'm also relieved to have my own space again. Being a couple is hard work."

Most of us hope to find our soul mate, but by the time we reach 30, life has made us a little more realistic about love. It isn't all effortless magic. We realize that a relationship takes time. Love just doesn't always happen. You have to work on it. There will be good times, but there will be tough times too. You just have to try and see if it works. The women I talked to who were in committed relationships admitted that at times it was not always easy, but they also spoke in glowing terms of the rewards. Mary, age 34, has just given birth to her baby boy. The bond between her and her husband is strong, but not without a struggle or two. "Leaving someone is far easier than trying to work things out," she says. "If a couple can talk about their problems and work something out that is mutually satisfying, that is the greatest joy of all."

Partnerships in the 30s tend to be richer and more complex than in the 20s. There may be a little less intensity, but if there is a commitment on both sides and both parties are prepared to compromise, grown-up love is not only calmer, but infinitely more rewarding.

There is something else that is also supposed to get better as we age—sex.

Sex in the 30s

"I'm waiting to hit the sexual peak I read about in all those magazines," says Mary, age 33. "A depressing card for my thirtieth birthday put a damper on things. It showed a group of men and women in a cable car. The men were going down and the women were going up. There was no meeting in between."

The cable car of course represented sex drive. Research has shown that women tend to enjoy sex more as they get older. Men's testosterone levels, however, are at their peak in their late teens. After that it's downhill all the way. This can cause relationship problems.

Almost all women in their 30s will have had experience not just of love, but of sex. Problems with our love life and with friendships can still be stressful, but many of us should feel more comfortable with our sexuality. Here's another one of nature's little tricks: When you start feeling more sexual your body starts going downhill. When your sexual prime kicks in society begins to lose interest.

Myths about sex and getting older continue to restrict and limit our self-expression: Women in their 30s are at their sexual peak. Older women shouldn't flaunt their sexuality. Pregnant women shouldn't have sex. Children ruin your sex life. One night stands aren't really appropriate when you are over 30.

I talked to countless women who disproved all these myths. It almost seems that getting satisfying sex in your 30s is all about moving away from such stereotypes.

You may have outgrown the sexual habits of your 20s. You may or may not want to have casual sex anymore. You may or may not be experiencing your sexual peak. Several women in their mid-30s wondered when exactly it would hit them. I also spoke to women who were perplexed by their loss of libido and others who had chosen celibacy. Whatever the state of your sex life, the important thing to remember is that just because you reach 30, you don't suddenly have to conform. Conformity is aging. You are an adult and should be capable of making your own choices and seeking out your own pleasure.

Tick Tock

In the 30s, the ticking biological clock often prompts us to make decisions. Grown-up decisions about settling down, finances, a house, and starting a family. Are we ready?

The decision to have a child is without a doubt one of the most important decisions you will ever make. The consequences of your decision will affect you for the rest of your life. All the women I talked to about motherhood, whether moms or not, had strong opinions about it. There were many doubts and fears. Many felt that motherhood would age them.

The reason we wrestle with the idea of motherhood in our 30s is obvious. Our bodies are reminding us that we are getting older. Women do give birth in their 40s, but our reproductive capacity is at its prime in our 20s and after that it begins to decline. The problem is that after sampling independence in our 20s many of us find the notion of being responsible for a child scary.

"Every time I work late or my boss sends me on a trip abroad or when I go to this wild party I am so glad that I have not got a kid," says Elizabeth, age 35. "I do want a kid but I need my life to be a bit more settled before I do that. I need a husband, a house, regular meals, and of course lots of money."

The decision to have a child is determined by so many factors. Is it the right time? Is my relationship stable? Will I get time off work? Can we afford this? What about my career goals?

But even when the pros outweigh the cons, is it a good time to have kids? "There never is a right time to have kids," says Nancy, age 37 and mother of two. "Lots of women wait until they are more financially stable and are well on their career path, but you have more energy when you are younger. Instead of spending your mid-life with teenage angst you can go off and do your own thing with your kids all grown up."

In her controversial new book, *What Our Mothers Didn't Tell Us: Why Happiness Eludes the Modern Woman* (1999), Danielle Crittenden argues that modern life has been "turned upside down" because women are delaying childbearing and women are losing out. She argues that we have "created a wasteland" of desperate singles, harassed mothers, miserable children, and overworked fertility experts.

Crittenden's argument is one-sided. It is indisputable that fertility does decline in the 30s, but the social and psychological factors argue against her. Older women know themselves better. They also tend to have established themselves financially and can take the time to enjoy their children growing up. At the end of the day one can't prescribe. There are pros and cons whatever age a woman decides to have a baby. It's a matter of each person's life script.

Some women decide that a family is not for them. Sally, age 32, had her tubes tied when she was 26. "I have no regrets about the decision I made at the time. I won't ever change my mind. Kids are not for me. People told me that I would regret it when I was in my thirties but I feel the same. There are so many children without loving families if I ever feel the need to mother I can always adopt. I just don't have the urge to have my own baby."

For some women in their 30s, motherhood is far from appealing. The popular notion that took root in the sixties, and that has lingered on, is that the world would grind to a halt if we did not stop reproducing soon. Our generation grew up with this kind of radical thinking. We may be haunted by the image of the perfect mom.

Many of us feel that we will never live up to it. Our moms too may have increased our doubts about this motherhood thing. "Giving birth to you and your brother was the most incredible experience, but I wish I had waited a few years until I had you. There was so much more I could have done with my life," Cindy, age 39, recalls her mother saying to her many times.

The messages about motherhood we may have received from our moms are confusing because their struggle was different from the struggles we have. In our moms' day it was a challenge to go out into the workplace. Now the challenge is to juggle home and the workplace successfully. As this is not always easy to do motherhood may sound less appealing. Even more unsettling is when we read of high profile women, like the president of Coca-Cola UK, who decided to resign to spend more time with her family.

A recent spate of novels have dramatized what is becoming a common conflict between the demands of work and the demands of home. Diana Appleyard's *Homing Instinct* is an examle. Attempting to surprise her children, career woman and thirtysomething mother Carrie arrives too late at the nursery and sees them being collected by their nanny. She sees a snapshot of her children's daily life where she plays no part. She feels "neither needed or wanted. A mother surplus to her children's requirements" (1999, p. 230).

Your mother was probably a mother when she was in her 30s. Even though women were in the workforce they were seen as wives and mothers first. You, on the other hand, were born into a generation of women who had far more choice over their lives. Your mom probably only got this choice after she had raised you. Our generation seems to have come to the conclusion that you have to get things done for yourself before you have kids. More and more of us are postponing children. And when you have kids you have to become a master juggler, balancing family and work with perfect skill. Some busy working moms like their lives organized that way, others don't. It all depends on whether you are doing what you want with your life.

Of the moms I spoke to, all agreed that the transition to motherhood had a huge impact. Some said that having children gave their lives more meaning. On occasion, a baby took the pressure off them at work, either because it put work into perspective, they decided to work fewer hours, or simply because they took time off to have and care for a baby. Some moms felt older.

"I never got my figure back after the twins. Being a mom has certainly aged me in other ways. I think like a mom now. I guess I'm more sensible." (Amanda, age 40)

"You go into this baby thing with eyes closed. Then as they pass this helpless bundle to you when you leave the hospital all of a sudden it dawns on you. This child is your responsibility. Its absolutely terrifying. I can tell you it made me grow up fast." (Rachel, age 30)

"My priorities have changed since I was a mom. I do feel older certainly." (Lyn, age 33)

But aren't kids supposed to keep us feeling young? "It all depends on how you cope with the stresses of parenthood," advises Mandy, age 37 and mother of two. "If you are in the baby stage of sleepless nights, baby blues and constant feeding, lack of sleep and fatigue could be the problems. If your children are older, worry about schools and colleges and day care can be stressful. Or if you had children very young you may have ambivalent feelings about them leaving home and how you will organize your life with them no longer being center stage."

Children will probably be very much dependent on you for emotional and financial support. "My advice to new moms," says Rachel, age 41 and mother of four, "is: Remember, one day your babies won't be babies anymore. They won't need you so much. Be prepared for that time so that it doesn't come upon you like a black hole. Enjoy motherhood but also cultivate your own interests and your own life."

Having children is a loaded issue. We realize that our lifestyle has to change. That there are things we ought to give up. That our time is no longer our own. Amy, age 34, told me: "I just didn't realize how lucky I was to have free time to do what I wanted. Now with three kids even just a few minutes to myself is luxury. I've forgotten what it's like to go to the restroom by myself."

But personal space, spontaneity, late nights, drinking, smoking, and our waistlines were not the only things that the women I spoke to worried about. The biggest concern seemed to be about identity. Becoming a mom. Losing a sense of themselves.

"I didn't feel like me anymore. I was Chloe's mom." (Lucy, age 38)

"I'm scared that I'd lose myself in my baby. I wouldn't want to do anything for myself anymore." (Victoria, age 31)

"I was worried nobody would take me seriously anymore when I had the kids." (Mandy, age 32)

While researching for this book I spoke to about a hundred thirtysomething moms. Single moms told me of their struggles to raise a child. How hard it was to go against social stereotypes. How hard it was to find time for themselves. Whether single or in a relationship, all the moms I spoke to agreed that the responsibility of mothering was huge. Some felt burdened, but others saw it as a kind of rebirth. Whatever the response, one thing is clear: motherhood brings many changes. Nothing is really ever the same again. Let's talk about a few of them.

Attitude to work may change. I talked to moms who said that having a baby put the crisis and challenges of work into perspective; priorities shift. Others said that work became even more important for a sense of self. Some intended to go back to work but found themselves unable to leave their baby when their maternity leave ended. A few said that they resented the fact that they had to go back to work for financial necessity. Several said that having a baby had made them rethink their career entirely. Others started new careers. Some decided to work from home. Whether working or staying at home, it was clear that feelings of guilt about working or not working figured strongly for both stay-at-home and working moms.

With a baby on the scene relationships will certainly change.

Moms said that they tended naturally to gravitate toward other moms for companionship and that often their old circle of friends diminished. Motherhood can also change relationships with parents and make a woman think about her own childhood and how the way she was brought up shaped her. Relationships with partners obviously changed. Now there are three to consider. Some moms missed the special times, but others said that the baby made the bond grow stronger.

Having a baby changed their bodies. How much it changed, though, depended on the individual—what they ate and how active they were. Many moms said that having a baby made them feel less inhibited about their bodies. Some said it made them more appreciative and accepting. They realized that we are not all meant to be a size eight. That their health and their baby's health were far more important than how much they weighed. Some moms said they felt more compassionate and less self-centered. For the first time in their lives they knew that without hesitation they would sacrifice their own life for the sake of someone else—their child.

Without a doubt, motherhood can change your body, your life, and your mind about a great many things, but don't romantically assume that just because a woman has a baby that all her attitudes will immediately change for the better. Plenty of women retain narrow attitudes after childbirth. Plenty of single women find ways to nurture. Mothering does not require children. It became clear from my conversations that what makes the difference is not just going through the biological process, but being open to the experience of motherhood, and paying intention to the changes that can enrich your life.

The motherhood question is an integral part of the "what do I want to do with my life?" crisis of the age 30 transition. That's why we think about it so much in our 30s. Here's what Laura, age 31, said: "I feel so ashamed of saying this. I mean, I have a successful career. Deep down though I just want children and a home. It took me a long time to understand this about myself though. I come from a very goal-oriented family and I thought I was the same." Jo, age 34, on the other hand, realized how important her work was to her when her partner asked her about kids. "I just knew that I couldn't stay at home full time and look after the kids. I'd miss working."

If you are in your early 30s and feeling anxious about childbirth, the advice of Dockett and Beck in *Facing 30* might prove helpful: "Keep in mind life expectancy is longer than it used to be. It seems urgent to deal with this now but you really do have the time" (p. 116). Women are having children later and later. But don't get too complacent, and bear in mind that as 40 draws near it is time to start making decisions about children.

And if you do get pregnant, don't go into a mad panic. Somehow moms cope. Time and time again when I talked to pregnant women and moms in their 30s, there were only a few who expressed an "I'm not ready" or a "Do I really want this?" or "I'm terrified" attitude. Instead there was a sense of peace and anticipation. An "I can handle it" attitude.

But what of those of us who do finally make the decision to have a baby in our 30s and then find that conception isn't as easy as we thought?

Nothing can be more aging in the 30s than the devastation and frustration of infertility.

No Baby

Statistically, one in six couples will have trouble having their own biological child. When a woman has put off having a child, hoping to get her career on track or because she didn't feel ready, her chances of infertility increase, not only because of stress, exposure to environmental toxins, and possibly hormonal problems, but because her eggs are getting older.

It is a cruel irony that after spending our teens and 20s trying not to get pregnant, some of us spend our 30s and 40s trying to have a child.

With modern fertility treatments, it is possible to have a baby in your 40s and even 50s, but these cases are quite rare and often achieved with a great deal of good luck. We just don't hear about all the unsuccessful patients of fertility treatments. And there are many of them. The stress of infertility treatment can lead to premature aging. Psychologist Alice D. Domar, director of the Women's Health Programs at the Mind/Body Institute of the New England Deaconess Hospital, found that women trying unsuccessfully to get pregnant have stress levels equivalent to women with cancer, HIV, and heart disease (Borysenko, *Woman's Book*, p. 106). And stress, according to many experts, makes infertility even more likely. Conception can become the main focus of their lives, putting them on a roller coaster ride that ends with dashed hopes once a month when their periods arrive. Tracking ovulation takes all the fun out of sex, and relationships suffer or break down.

Work: "And What Do You Do?"

The way you choose to earn a living tends to become a label. This is even more apparent in your 30s, when the expectation is that you will be settling down into a career. Sandy, age 33, says that she always suffers terribly at parties. Whenever she mentions that she is a housewife she can see eyes glaze over. She becomes forgettable. Rachel, age 37, on the other hand, admits that her career as a prison warden has not hindered but helped her social life. Men and women always seem to be fascinated by her choice of job.

According to Lauren Dockett and Kristin Beck in *Facing 30*, the work you do in your 30s becomes a kind of "tidy category . . . a key of sorts to understanding who the multifaceted woman you once were has settled down to become" (p. 59). The really scary part of all this is that for some of us a job is no longer something you do in order to earn a living, it is dangerously close to becoming, in other people's minds, something you are. "It was frightening," says Nancy, age 31. "When I say I work for women's magazines, people get this idea of me which isn't true at all. There is a part of me that wants to do something real, something genuine, and get away from all this superficial stuff."

Like many of us in our early 30s who may be at a worker's crossroads, Nancy is undecided about her future career plans. If we are going to get the fulfilling career, now is the time. The fear is that before you know it you will have joined the rat race and become like millions of others. The 30s are about not just finding the rewarding career that also pays the bills, but about getting on the right path. Many of us long to find our life task. To find a job that is fulfilling and rewarding. It can be frustrating to still feel you are searching, and every time you are asked what you do your incoherent reply seems like an admission of failure. There is such pressure to act like a working adult. Much of this pressure, though, is put upon us ourselves. We think that once a decision has been made we can't alter it. It is more difficult to change when you are in your 30s, but part of the maturing process of adulthood is understanding that life is a series of choices, and what you do is only a part of who you are. People are far too complex and multifaceted to be defined by their careers, especially in this age when career change is the norm. Just because you are doing something in your 30s does not mean that you will be doing it for the rest of your life.

Still, it can be depressing if you don't seem to be getting anywhere. Tracy, age 32, is an aspiring singer. She has been close to two record deals, but they have both fallen through. To pay the rent, she works in an all-night café. What seemed carefree and exciting in her 20s is starting to become tiring and humiliating in her 30s. "I've looked into many careers, but at the end of the day nothing seems to inspire me except music. I'm getting older though. I want to be treated with a little more dignity." In contrast to Tracy, there are many women in their 30s who are, in the eyes of the world, well on the track. Their careers are flourishing. Curiously, though, when asked many said that they longed to be irresponsible again. To have a job without deadlines when everything didn't depend on them.

Whatever the work dilemma, most of us will by now have different expectations about work. We may still not know what we want to do, but at least we know what we definitely don't want to do.

When I talked to thirtysomething women about their careers, it was clear that even though incredible advances had been made there was still a long way to go before women felt there was total equality alongside men. But despite this, a lot of positive messages about work did come through. Working environment, challenge, and learning something new often seemed more important than prestige, high salaries, and your own office for many women. The workplace has many negatives, especially in this age of specialization, but most of the women I talked to were starting to feel satisfied. A few said that money was the motivating factor, but many more said that although the money was great it didn't really change their lives that much. Job satisfaction was key. Others said that they were getting better at finding balance between work and leisure.

On the whole it became apparent that work in the 30s was all about finding out that you can do more than you thought you could. The 30s is the decade, not of conformity and keeping on track, but of new possibilities.

Relationships and Social Life

"When I was at college I had hundreds of friends. My birthday parties were huge. The phone was always ringing. Now that I'm in my thirties, that doesn't happen anymore. I have about three good friends I know I can rely on. The trouble with knowing lots and lots of people is that you never really get to know them well and that can make conversations quite tedious." (Deborah, age 34)

A hallmark of the 30s is a closer circle of friends. Maturity and growing self-confidence often bring discrimination in friendships. You don't feel the need to be around so many people all the time. And it's not just the number of your friends that change. The nature of your relationships change.

"Now I'm getting older and hopefully a bit more mature, I don't need to see my friends all the time and I don't expect too much from them. Those days when you did everything together are long since over. We all have our own lives to lead and we all have different interests." (Raine, age 36)

In your 30s, when you have a clearer sense of your need for companionship and the needs of others, friendship does change in nature, but bonds can also grow stronger. "When I broke up with my boyfriend on my thirtieth birthday," says Kathryn, "I don't know what I would have done without my friends. They nursed me through the bad times and gave me my self-confidence back. I wouldn't hesitate to do the same for any one of them."

Getting to your 30s can also be a defining moment for your relationship with your family. It may suddenly dawn on you that it's time to stop blaming your parents for everything. You may find yourself drifting away or coming closer. You may even stop trying to make them see things your way and accept them for what they are. I have always had a difficult relationship with my father. Part of me blamed him for the early death of my mother. Another resented the fact that he was never there for us, could never hold down a job. We used to have terrible arguments when I was growing up. It got to the point when I couldn't be in the same room as he. I didn't see him for most of my 20s. In my 30s we see each other occasionally. It's okay between us now. He doesn't upset me anymore. I see him for what he is. I don't expect anything from him.

As far as social life in the 30s is concerned, it's there if you want it. I talked to women who always seemed to be partying and those who rarely went out. Neither was more content than the other. The only ones who seemed apprehensive about their social lives were the ones who were still in the "staying in on a Saturday night has to be the most depressing thing that can happen to you" mindset. The 30s offer liberation from that mindset. You realize that it is not just old people and people with no friends who don't go out all the time, but people like yourself who might prefer to relax at home and enjoy their own company.

Balancing our need for connection with our need for being an individual is one of the greatest psychological stresses for the 30s. The 30s can bring with them a new kind of clarity, honesty, and self-assertion. "You know who you want to be around," says Rachel, age 35. "Some of my friends were like black holes. They sucked away all my energy. Now I don't want to be with them anymore. I want to be around people who bring the good out in me. Hopefully I bring the good out of them too." Nina, age 37, feels similarly. "I want to be honest in my relationships. I don't want to play games anymore or be someone I'm not. I want there to be give and take. I just want to be me and not be judged all the time."

Self-Esteem—Am I Grown Up Now?

"Today," writes Gail Sheehy in *New Passages*, "the transition to the Turbulent Thirties marks the initiation to First Adulthood . . . Americans today do not become adults until their late twenties" (p. 59).

Fifty years ago, age 30 was responsible and grown up. But life patterns have changed. We can be kids for longer. Take more time over our education. Start families later. We can change careers because the job market is flexible. We can travel. We don't have to settle down right after school. The breakdown of the family unit and high divorce rates means that we haven't grown up with traditional ideas about family, work, and love anymore. We know that we have choices.

"Just because someone has a family, a job, and a house doesn't automatically mean that they are happy. Adult fulfillment is much more complex than that." (Mary, age 35)

"I want to know more about myself before I go for all that. It's tragic when you see people doing things for the wrong reasons and finding out later when something traumatic happens. I don't want to be like that." (Carla, age 33)

Women in their 30s have been exposed to a lot about the adult world. We may even be disillusioned. We know that our parents didn't necessarily have all the answers. That growing up is about much more than settling down, marriage, and kids. Many of us are taking our time "growing up." Finding out what we want. This kind of experimentation is associated with the 20s, when we try on personalities like hats.

Extended adolescence in the 30s is becoming increasingly common. The older generation may call it escapism, but perhaps our lack of enthusiasm for commitment to a path is, in this day and age, a wiser choice. We are learning, taking our time, feeling our way. We don't want to end up lost, like so many of our parents are.

"I'm not ready for the house, car, and 2.4 children yet. I haven't yet met anyone I want to share my life with and I'm still determined to make something of my artwork. I'm not giving up yet. I'm still not sure what I want out of life. Some days I think I'll just pack my bags and go traveling around the world." (Becky, age 33)

Whether or not we are finding focus in our 30s, most of us won't *feel* 30. We are still changing interests and interpretations, but it is important to realize that in the course of our adult development none of this is wasted. Gail Sheehy's advice in *Passages* (1976) is useful. She reminds us that action, trying out new things, and experimenting is healthy during the 20s and early 30s. "Introspection is a dangerous thing," if it interferes with action. All the choices we make inform our course for the future and increase our self-knowledge. We may not know it now, but one day we will look back and understand that everything we did in our lives served a purpose. There is no such thing as a wasted experience. All we were doing was finding out what our interests are and what we want to be.

This, of course, is something we only truly learn in retrospect. The cruel truth is that right now all we know is how disheartening a blow it is to our self-esteem to be in our 30s and to feel that we haven't achieved much. The misconception that by the age of 30 you should be doing grown-up things and have achieved your life's ambition can be very frustrating. Frustration is an aging emotion.

You may feel that you should be impressed with yourself now, or that society should have recognized your achievements in some way. Childhood passions return to haunt you like the ghost of Christmas past. Weren't you supposed to have done this or that by now? Weren't you going to be famous? What about that novel you were going to write? Weren't you supposed to be on the board of directors by now? What about marriage and children? What about that Ph.D.?

The age 30 transition is not always a smooth ride. Letting go of your old life and trying to create a new one with only what you know you don't like as a guide can be frightening and frustrating. "When I was ten I had my life figured out," says Mary-Ann. "I was going to go to college, have a job, and then start a family. I didn't know that I would discover I had a talent for acting and throw myself wholeheartedly into that. I'm thirty-four now and thinking about going back to college after dropping out when I was eighteen. I'm scared of making the wrong decision again."

Part of growing up in the 30s is watching our childhood fantasies die, and re-evaluating our lives as they are now. They don't match our grown-up selves anymore. "It wasn't until I reached thirty," says Natasha, age 31, "that I finally abandoned my dream of being a famous model. Now I realize that I wasn't really suited for the life anyway." On the other hand, for those of us who have achieved our goals early there may be the depressing realization that this isn't exactly what we wanted, that our lives aren't really making us happy. "I had everything I thought I wanted at thirty. A glamorous job, lots of money, and a boyfriend, but I was miserable. Life still seemed difficult," says Lara, age 36.

As well as apprehension about the life choices we have made, the 30s may also bring with them regret that we weren't as wild as we could have been. "I regret that I didn't just have more fun my twenties. I didn't sleep around much. I was too shy to go to parties. I've stuck with the same job. I feel like I haven't lived," says Lana, age 32. In your 20s, doing wild, crazy things is almost expected; in your 30s you and everyone else knows that you are old enough to know better. For those of us who did act crazy when we were younger there was little regret, but an acknowledgment that the time to do so was past; that in the 30s and 40s it was time to "sober up" a little—not to stop dead in our tracks, but to think a little more about our responsibilities before we act.

Experts in human development talk about the process of mastery, through which individuals achieve a kind of wisdom—they know what they can control in their lives and what they cannot; they learn to let go. In our 30s we are caught in the middle of two phases (the questioning of the 20s and the acceptance of later life when we try to problem-solve and work with what is). The fear and anxiety of the early 30s can perhaps be explained by the fact that we are at a crossroads, and have these contradictory instincts. "I still want to travel a lot," says Mary, age 33, "but not quite as much as before. I don't want to settle down but I do want some sort of stability."

Learning to live your life in a way that is different from your youthful ambitions can feel like letting yourself down. But appreciating why you gave up these dreams and what they have taught you about yourself will help you create new ones that suit you more now. The "by now" crisis of the 30s that Gail Sheehy describes as "a vague but persistent sense of wanting to be something more" (*Passages*, p. 198) can help us focus on our dreams with the eye of someone who knows a bit more about the world and about ourselves. Childhood dreams, which depended on our innocence to be realized, may have to abandoned or modified in some way, but at least now you can begin to formulate a new plan for your life as an adult.

You might find it depressing that in your 30s starting a new life plan, new projects, joining new clubs and societies, and learning a new skill may not have the same feeling of promise and opportunity. Instructors and employers may not view you with quite so much enthusiasm. It can be hard not to feel that your time has passed and that of the younger generation has begun, that whatever you do now won't have quite the same meaning. "There's still a lot I want to do," says Linda, age 34, "but when it comes to it I feel ridiculous starting something new. I could never be one of these women who goes back to college or something like that. The time for all that has passed."

Too many of us, like Linda, put limitations on ourselves in the 30s. True, our lives may be more structured and busy due to family or career, but the only person stopping us from starting new projects is ourselves. Although youthful ambitions may have to be modified according to life circumstances, there is no law that says starting something new or learning something new in the 30s is inappropriate. In fact, women who see every day as a learning experience tend to be the ones who are more youthful and vital. Those that believe they are "too old for this" and "too old for that" accelerate the aging process.

Many women agreed that it wasn't until the 30s approached that they could actually formulate a plan for their lives, because only now were they beginning to make sense of themselves and where their interests lay. It's not really until your 30s that you start to know yourself a little better and can finally be in a position to make changes or form new plans. Rebecca, age 33, realized as she approached 30 that she had simply become a teacher because her parents had always thought she would. She never felt right in a classroom. Currently she is in the fourth year of a five-year medical training course.

Like Rebecca, many women found that the 30s involved being less pressured by the opinions of others and the demands of the moment, and being more true to yourself. Tilsner assures her readers in *29 and Counting* that turning 30 is the last time you are burdened down with adolescent angst about what other people think. "The whole turning 30 trauma is the last, dramatic flare up of such urges" (p. 131). Sometime in your early 30s you stop comparing yourself to others, you stop worrying about what others expect of you. You start living your life the way you want it. You start building your self-esteem. And, boy, can that be liberating!

"I thought I knew what I wanted in my twenties," says Sasha, age 37, "but I didn't really have a clue. I was still finding my way.

Learning about myself. I was also desperately insecure and too willing to please. I wouldn't want to go back to those days. It's much more exciting being older, more in control of my life."

Looking Older: You've Hit 30 and It Looks like It's Hit You

In your 30s, bodily complaints put you in touch with the reality of aging as never before. You may even find yourself listing them in a voice that reminds you of your mother, or your grandmother. "I'll give you a list of the things that bother me," says Jane, age 30. "Fatigue, aches and pains, PMS, thinning nails, and cellulite." "I've got dry skin and wrinkles, and I can't lose weight as quickly because my body has made friends with my fat," adds Jennifer, age 36. "My back aches more," says Rebecca, at 38. "I'm not as toned as I used to be. I keep forgetting things. My hair is getting thinner. I thought I wouldn't have to deal with this until I was at least fifty."

Symptoms of aging in your 30s may come as an unhappy surprise. Like Rebecca, you may have thought you wouldn't have to deal with this until you were in your 50s. For the first time many of us see our faces and our bodies begin to change. We get to know our doctors better. We hear more and more about people getting sick and dying. We see our parents getting frailer.

We still live in a culture obsessed with youth. "The message we get from the day we are born is clear: youth, beauty, and money rank above all else in our culture" (Tilsner, p. 18). Giving up that youth can be daunting, almost like a loss of power. It's not just about being fresh-faced and firm anymore, but about feeling that we are moving to the sidelines, fading from color to black and white. Perfect looks and young beauty have been our role models. Now they simply remind us that we are getting older.

Getting older can make some of us fiercely critical about our bodies. Diet, exercise, and beauty routines become very important.

Some of us may be more accepting, but even so it's difficult not to feel disappointed with your body as 30 approaches. "It's harder to like your body," says Monica, age 33. "I'm not twenty-one anymore, that's for sure. . . . I take longer to heal and my bones ache. I have a few wrinkles and even the odd gray hair. My breasts are less firm, and my tummy has a soft spot since I had my baby. I can't act wild like I used to."

Some women said that reaching 30 and looking older was a relief. They felt more honest and realistic about their bodies. They could put the insecurity of the 20s behind them. "I don't hate my thighs anymore. I deal with them," says Kristin, age 34. "I used to stay away from the beach 'cause I thought I looked terrible in a swimsuit. I don't do those kind of things anymore. Life is too short."

But even those apparently carefree about bodily aging felt a pang of regret that their visibility was not so high. As we start to view our bodies and our lives differently, we might notice that others do, too. Linda, age 33, made this comment about her changing looks "When I was twenty and I walked down the street I got comments and screams from cars. Now I'm thirty-six and it's happening less and less. I'm relieved but it does make me think about how much my body has changed."

We are all annoyingly aware of the double standard. Men get sexier as they age, while women past the age of about 32 simply get old. Just think of all those Hollywood May-to-December pairings when aging stars like Sean Connery and Michael Douglas play alongside young female stars who could be their daughters or even granddaughters. There are signs, however, that this is beginning to change and that the age limit for women is edging up. Cher and Susan Sarandon are examples of mature beauty and glamour.

Princess Diana was 37 when she died, yet everyone agrees she was in the prime of her beauty. This made her death all the more poignant. Our generation mourned her for many reasons, and one of them was because we lost the opportunity to watch her grow old with us. In the words of Dr. Priscilla Stuckey, a bookcrafter and women's health expert, "We lost a companion in aging. With her early death she will always remain young in the eyes of the world, so she won't be revising everyone's opinion of beauty and age, but many of us felt years older when she died. As if she carried our youth, our prime, away with her."

We know that the "youth equals beauty" equation is a cultural construction, and that for many women, the prime of their lives is in their later years, but it still doesn't make visible signs of aging any easier to live with. Aging brings us face to face with our own mortality. The fragility of life definitely becomes apparent. Maybe a friend develops breast cancer, or your mom, who is clearly aging, requires special attention. Your own early signs of aging remind you that you too are getting older and that eventually your body will wear out.

Coming to terms with being 30 is in many ways like coming to terms with death itself. Expect to go through all the five stages of grieving for the loss of your youth—fear, denial, anger, bargaining, and eventually, acceptance.

The chances are that in your 30s someone dear to you will have passed away. It is important to grieve and to respect the memory of the loved one, but prolonged grieving is unhealthy and aging. In some cultures death is something to be celebrated, not mourned. If a partner or a loved one dies, seeing a young woman become haunted and haggard and obsessed with the past is cause for concern. People can and have died from a broken heart. Sometimes it can be the final straw and all will to live is lost. But it is important to remember that we are meant to live life to the fullest, that life goes on. To perpetually grieve is to be antilife. And to be antilife is to imply that not only your life, but the lives of those departed, were worthless too.

Coming to terms with death and loss can make you look and feel younger. When my mother died in my late 20s, I was an emotional wreck, but I allowed myself to have all the emotions I needed to have—from anger to self-pity. After years of emotional fragility and crying more than not crying, the balance finally shifted. In my 30s, I realized that lots of the old conflicts had been shifted through grieving. I got my vibrancy back. Accepting the reality of death need not age and depress you. It can mature you and help you look and feel younger, happier, and more vital than ever before.

We lose many things as we age—from our youthful bodies to our youthful aspirations. Death not only refers to the loss of a loved one, but to the loss of anything that you valued and that gave your life meaning. The loss of a job or the end of a relationship can be like a kind of death. All these "deaths" can be traumatic if we allow them to be. It all depends on our response. Hopefully, time will teach us that getting older means loss of all kinds. It is up to us to come to terms with the reality of death and loss and, after a mourning period, to move forward with our lives.

We may regret that we have to say goodbye to our youthful bodies, but our changing bodies can encourage us to make a renewed commitment to treating ourselves better. "I know I can't live on junk food and a few hours of sleep anymore. My body has its limitations. I have to be more careful," says Anna, age 36. The recognition that we need to start being more careful with our bodies may make us feel older, but it can also usher in a time to start taking better care of ourselves. It can bring the realization that good health is the most valuable asset we have, and if we want our bodies to age well we are going to have to treat them with more respect.

Having looked at some of the challenges we face in our 30s, let's now explore some of the various explanations offered for the underlying sense of crisis and transition many of us feel when we hit 30—regardless of whether love, work, family, friends, sex, bodily change, or self-esteem is the big issue in our lives at present.

Chapter 3
The Age 30 Transition

Linda married when she was 22, right after college. Two children later, at the age of 30, she is ready to begin a new phase in her life. She is hopeful about her future. "There is so much I want to do now that the kids are in school. I want to teach. I wouldn't have been ready at twenty-two but I am now."

Sarah, age 31, is also excited about the transition. "I love being in my thirties. In my twenties I felt like a reed blown in the wind. I followed in the direction of everyone else. I don't want to do that anymore. I now realize that what I think matters."

In contrast to Linda and Sarah, many of us might feel more empathy with Robin, age 30, who isn't so positive about becoming 30. "I don't know what I want. I still have this longing to see the world. I don't feel ready to settle down into a routine just yet. But there are times when I think it would be nice to have my own apartment and a steady relationship. I feel like two people at the moment. One moment a child, the next an adult. It doesn't help that all my friends are just as stressed about reaching thirty as I am. It's horrible."

Developmental psychologists of our generation have offered an explanation for the anxiety many of us feel about the 30s. They think of the late 20s to the early 30s as a time of change and transition from childhood to adulthood. A time of restlessness when new choices must be made. "The work involves great change, turmoil, and commonly crisis—a simultaneous feeling of rock bottom and the urge to break out" (Sheehy, *Passages*, p. 199).

Daniel Levinson, a Yale psychologist and author of *The Seasons of a Woman's Life* (1996), describes these years as the "age 30 transition." Life, according to Levinson, is a series of transitions, and these periods are often times of crisis. The transit time occurs between the end of one life phase and the structures we have grown familiar with, and the beginning of another life phase when we start to build something new. Levinson suggests that approaching 30 brings with it a re-evaluation and assessment of all that we did in the 20s so that we can enter the first fully adult decade with a new agenda and, hopefully, with renewed confidence.

Psychologists may be able to analyze why many of us feel ill at the thought of turning 30, but it's obvious why we are panicking. We are not in our 20s anymore. We have no idea what to expect. We find it impossible to see in the future while we are in the crisis. More is expected of us from family, community, and society. We wonder if we will still be desirable in a culture that assigns beauty and hireability to youth. To find personal fulfillment we need to bring some kind of focus to our lives at a time when we are anything but focused. Considering the pressure, it is no surprise that many women, like Mary, age 33, face anxiety and depression in the late 20s as 30 draws closer and closer.

"In my late twenties, the depression started. I had everything I thought I wanted. My career was on track. I had my own place and an active social life. But I wasn't happy at all. It got to the point that my weekends would be spent in bed. I just didn't have any enthusiasm for anything anymore. I started seeing a therapist the week after my thirtieth birthday."

Psychologists and doctors I talked to often said that many of their female patients start seeing therapists in their 30s. According to Levinson, depression around age 30 is related to issues from childhood that remain unresolved. Somehow during the 20s we carry on. There is a lot we know we need to work on but the resilience and hope of youth helps us get by. By the age of 30 we lose a bit of our resilience. We understand that age does not necessarily bring with it wisdom. That if we don't sort ourselves out nobody else will. That everybody doesn't live happily ever after. That depression and fear are becoming harder and harder to hide. We need to envision a life for us that is appropriate for the 30s, and not the 20s. The sense of crisis and anxiety that comes with age 30 forces us to take a long, hard look at ourselves. It's like a wake-up call for us to face up to who we are and what we want out of life. For some of us this may be too painful to do alone and we may need help from therapists.

Developmental Stages in a Woman's Life

My own need to understand more about my own feelings of anxiety and crisis in my early 30s and why so many thirtysomething women get depressed led me to research all the developmental stages in a woman's life. What holds us back and what helps us mature? How does one phase in life prepare for the next? What is this angst about being 30 all about?

Initially what struck me was not just the lack of information about developmental stages in a woman's life, but the failure of medical science and psychology to consider women in their own right and not as pseudo-men. Women and men do share the same characteristics. We are more alike than we are dissimilar. But the characteristics of the female life cycle do have distinct differences from the characteristics of the male life cycle and deserve more serious attention.

As I researched I began to notice an interesting development. Joan Borysenko highlights this in her commendable study of the female life cycle *A Woman's Book of Life: The Biology, Psychology, and Spirituality of the Feminine Life Cycle* (1996). From traditions as varied as the work of C. G. Jung, the Bible, the Native American tradition, Buddhist law, and astrology, Borysenko points out that a "seven year cycle" as a reference for the human life cycle keeps reappearing.

The chakra system, which employs a system of sevens for understanding the human body, its energy centers, and phases of development, is a case in point. Chakras, the body's energy centers, are thought to influence our spiritual and physical well-being and are often described as "whirling pools" of energy. They run from the base of your spine to the top of your head, each represented by a color, sound, element, and set of emotions. Each chakra is also responsible for a stage in our spiritual and physical development and governs different systems in our body.

The 30s are governed by the third eye and crown chakras. Insight, perception, and fulfillment are the positives, depression and anxiety the negatives. One stage of development begins in the last years of the 20s and ends in the mid-30s. Many of the women I talked to confirmed that just before their thirtieth birthday and then again in their middle to late 30s there was a great deal of restlessness and change in their lives.

Ancient Chinese philosophy employs a similar system of seven-year cycles for understanding the body and how it parallels the workings of the universe. Unfortunately, men are supposed to grow in wisdom and maturity, while women just grow old and useless sexually.

According to these ancient traditions, life can be divided into seven-year cycles. Every seven years, changes occur that are both visible and invisible. Cells are replaced in the body and physical growth, mental growth, and emotional growth occur. Seen in this light the crises of the late 20s and the mid-30s are just a normal part of the life cycle. In every life cycle there are many markers and turning points, and turning 30 is one of them.

Astrologically, I found another thought-provoking explanation for the 30s being a particularly stressful period of life. This is the theory of the Saturn return. Every 30 years or so Saturn returns to the same position on your birth chart as it did when you were born. Saturn represents a time of limitation. It can bring with it depression and frustration, but viewed positively it can be a time for making an honest assessment of progress made so far and choices for the future.

Not being an expert on the chakras, astrology, or ancient philosophies, I searched elsewhere for information about the developmental stages in a woman's life. Even though I did find some theories by developmental psychologists about life stages, everywhere it was the same. Where the female life cycle and physiological aging in a woman have been studied, it has traditionally been limited by its reference to our reproductive life.

All the emphasis has been placed on the maiden (desirability), mother (productivity), and crone (undesirability) explanations of the female life cycle. Adolescence, childbirth, and menopause were explored, examined, and outlined in detail. A century ago this may have made sense. Children were vulnerable and many died young. If a girl survived childhood diseases the next biggest threat to her life would be childbirth. Today, however, the female life cycle needs updating. A woman is no longer defined by the use she makes of her reproductive organs. Her life is no longer dictated by the needs of her family.

In the great majority of cases, psychological and emotional crises specific to the late 20s and mid-30s were either brief or omitted altogether. It was a similar story when I researched physiological change in the 30s. The 30s are rarely mentioned.

On the whole, medical science and psychology have neglected the many and varied phases in a woman's life, but there are notable exceptions. It was encouraging when I researched popular nonfiction to find that attention is finally being paid to the age 30 transition. Written by women in their 30s for women approaching 30, studies like *Facing 30* by Lauren Dockett and Kristin Beck and *29 and Counting* by Julie Tilsner explore the age 30 angst with insight and wit. But even though I thoroughly enjoyed these handbooks, I did feel that the focus was always on the early 30s and not the decade as a whole. There wasn't enough information about bodily aging in the 30s, how this affects every area of your life, and how to cope with it.

Extremely helpful in my research was the work of Gail Sheehy. In her groundbreaking book, *Passages*, she was one of the first to bring public attention to the many predictable crises in adult life. Using case histories of women and men of all ages, she explored in detail the mysteries of the life cycle. Typical rites of passage that face men and the different rites of passage that women encounter are examined. Originally intending to write a book about mid-life crisis, she found herself drawn into a subject infinitely more complex. "There were crises all along, or rather points of turning," she notes.

Sheehy's book attempted to show readers how they could use each life crisis as an opportunity for creative change—to grow into their full potential. Her road map of adult life explored the inevitable personality and sexual changes we go through in our 20s, 30s, 40s, and beyond. After the "Trying 20s," when the safety of home is left behind, we begin trying on life's uniforms in search of the perfect fit. A section is devoted to "Catch 30," when illusions are shaken and it's time to break or deepen life commitments.

Because it was among the first to navigate uncharted waters, *Passages* was an instant success. It helped many people make better sense of the transitions that they experience in their lives from teenage to old age. Unfortunately, though, for those of us in our 30s at the beginning of the millennium, the book has lost its relevance. In the last 20 years, a historic revolution has occurred in the adult life cycle. In the 1990s young people are leaving home later, and more women postpone having children until their 30s or 40s. People are taking longer to grow up and much longer to grow old. Predictable life crises are very different now than those our parents faced.

In Sheehy's updated version, *New Passages*, she acknowledges that the 30s mark the initiation into first adulthood, when "prolonged adolescence ends . . . when we are not afraid to disappoint our parents," but the main focus of the book is the "flourishing 40s" and the "flaming 50s."

Although Sheehy's *Passages* is dated and does not fully address bodily aging, it helped me understand more clearly the crisis women experience in their 30s. My research also led me to other outstanding contributions to the study of the female life cycle.

Extraordinarily insightful was Joan Borysenko's *A Woman's Book of Life*. Following the guidance of ancient philosophies, the periods of a woman's life are divided into 12 seven-year periods, three in each quadrant of life—childhood and adolescence, young adulthood and mid-life, and the later years. Issues pertaining to each cycle are explored in turn. The study is unique in that it explores not just psychological and emotional change, but bodily change for women of all ages, proposing that it is impossible to discuss one without mention of the other two.

Also helpful was Daniel Levinson's *The Seasons of a Woman's Life*. Levinson used the same theory of other great developmental psychologists like Erik Erikson. He interviewed 45 women at various life stages, and after 15 years came up with keen assessments about the female life cycle from the teens to the 40s. Levinson makes the point that part of growing up is seeing your old life structures go into decline and putting new ones in place to suit the next phase in your life. Life structures are our hopes and our dreams, how we fit into the world, what is important to us and what makes us happy. The early 30s, according to Levinson are what he calls a "transition period" when structures change.

Borysenko, Sheehy, and Levinson all agree that there is never any one crisis point in a woman's life, but rather a series of crises that seem to occur with predictable regularity. Some crisis points receive more attention than others. Menopause, for instance, is a huge transition, but it is no more or less important than other transitions that occur throughout our lives. Each stage in life has its challenges. During these transitional periods we question ourselves, and by going through them we emerge with a stronger sense of our own identity.

Life, then, is a series of turning points. The crises of the 30s is a stage on our life path. But I'm sure that any woman approaching or in her 30s would agree that because the age 30 transition is our first encounter with our adult selves, the turning point is a particularly compelling and interesting one to examine.

The 30s bring with them a number of psychologically and emotionally aging challenges—re-examining the hopes and expectations of our 20s; making decisions about work, family, marriage, and children; and coming to terms with the gradual loss of youth. Let's take a brief look at the two seven-year periods that define this decade of transition. Remember, though, that some of us mature earlier than others and the typical challenges we can expect to face will all be experienced in our own unique way.

Ages 28 to 35: Crisis and Change

The biggest issue facing women turning 30, it seems, is letting go of old routines and structures of the 20s and preparing to explore new possibilities.

Of the many women I interviewed for this book who were in this age bracket almost all confessed that their life was in some kind of crisis. There were decisions to be made. Should I leave my job? Should I think about a new career? Do I want children? Can I have children? Should I get divorced? Will I ever get married? How long will I stay looking young? Frequently, changes are made in their lives. Relationships ended. Housewives went back to college. Working moms found alternative arrangements for childcare. Those that were dissatisfied in their marriage divorced.

According to Levinson, the age 30 transition period, when we re-examine the life structures of our teens and 20s, spans the years between 28 and 32. Part of this re-examination is questioning what we really want from life. Do we want a career? Do we want a family? Do we want to get married? What is it that we as women want?

In Victorian times a woman was supposed to want to be plump and comforting for her husband and her children. According to Freud she was supposed to want to be a man. In the 1950s we were supposed to want to be housewives. In the 1960s we were supposed to want to burn our bras. In the 1970s we were supposed to want sex, drugs, and a carefree lifestyle. In the 1980s we were supposed to want to have a career. In the 1990s we were supposed to be able to achieve it all: a great body, a dazzling career, lots of money, a fantastic marriage, and beautifully behaved children.

As Joan Borysenko wrote, "The problem, of course, was cutting all women out of the same piece of cloth" (*Woman's Book*, p. 102). Generalizations and common assumptions about women's lives and what we are supposed to want are often woefully inadequate. We are not the same. Each one of us is different, with a different body, mind, and spirit. Some of us prefer to stay single. Others want to get married. Some of us want to have careers. Others want both career and marriage. No one life story will match everyone. Not every woman who goes to work and has children will feel exhausted. Not every woman who stays at home with her children will necessarily feel unfulfilled.

So the answer to the question, "What do women want?" is impossible to answer. Every woman has different needs and wants. It is during the age 30 transition, however, that for many of us the question "What do I want?" assumes a new urgency.

The age 30 crisis forces us to think about how we want to live and what is important to us. Hopefully, this will inspire us to make changes in our lives—so that rather than living lives that worked for us in our 20s but don't work now because our life circumstances are different, we can move on with a sense of excitement and optimism to the next phase of our lives. We can enter the first adult decade and step fully into our evolving selves. We can start learning about ourselves and what is important to us. We can start finding some kind of balance in our lives. We can start thinking about our legacy to the future.

And nothing gives us a sense of more urgency in the 30s than our biological clocks. Most women in their 30s admitted that the sense of crisis they felt in their 30s was directly related to the ticking of the biological clock: That marriage or not, children or not, more children or not, and how this would affect their life, their work, and their relationships was never far from their minds. It affected every decision they made.

We know that once we hit 30 we haven't got time on our hands. Levinson's studies reveal that at the onset most women with careers had similar life plans: career, marriage, children, resume, career. Many of them, however, had divorced or were still not married by their early 30s. A significant number of the women who were single and child-less admitted that the thought of never having a baby or never getting married was stressful. If we want to have children and haven't, the 30s are crunch time. We can decide to have children, or we can decide to nurture in other ways and concentrate on other aspects of our lives.

And for those women who did manage to have children and a career, there was another source of stress—the struggle between supermom and supercareer woman. But it's not just moms with careers that feel their lives are too crowded. Many of the women I talked to in their early 30s found that, for a variety of reasons from establishing a career to completing studies, there wasn't enough time for everything anymore. The greatest struggle for them is to find some kind of balance in their lives.

Age 35 to 42: Becoming an Adult

At 37, Rachel was a woman who had it all. A good figure, a great job as a magazine editor, three children, and a loving husband. But Rachel wasn't happy. In order to achieve so much she had been forced to become very organized. Sometimes she would look in her diary and get incredibly depressed. There was no room for spon-taneity in her life anymore. She knew exactly what was going to happen every minute of the day.

Rachel feels that the quality of her life is deteriorating. She can't understand why, because she feels she is achieving all that she wanted. She blames herself and feels guilty about being depressed.

In the late 30s and early 40s, with the age transition behind us, many women find themselves asking if they really enjoy their lives. According to Borysenko, between the ages of 35 and 42 major issues become more and more important: taking care of unfinished business from the past, which involves healing emotional wounds and thinking about how we live our lives. If we can do these successfully we stand a terrific chance of entering mid-life as satisfied and fulfilled women. "Making new priorities and completing prior developmental phases that we may not yet have fully mastered" are the two major rites of passage we face in the middle to late 30s (Borysenko, *Woman's Book*, p. 120).

The big question in the late 30s is, "Has anything been learned from the age thirty crisis?" Changes may have been made. Relationships may have begun or ended. Careers may have progressed or delayed. However, if nothing has been learned from our past, we won't be ready to become an adult. And if we haven't matured, unresolved issues tend to resurface and express themselves in emotional immaturity until we can find some way to deal with them positively.

Every kind of relationship we have, whether it be with husband, lover, friend, parent, or sibling, changes and develops. When a woman matures and becomes more sure of herself and what she wants, she begins to question the authenticity of many of her relationships. Marianne is 39 and has been divorced three times. Each marriage has ended amicably and she lives comfortably on the settlements. Recently she has noticed a change within herself. Finding a husband is no longer at the top of her list of priorities. In fact she's not altogether sure she is cut out for marriage at all. She's not ready to share her life again.

Time and time again, women in their 30s told me that this is the decade when they find out who their true friends are and who they do and don't want in their lives. Not surprisingly, the peak divorce rate for women is between the late 20s and early 30s. However, divorce rates continue to be high for women throughout their 30s.

By the end of our young adulthood we are ready to end relationships that are not mutually enhancing. Laura met Sally when they were both finishing college. They had shared the same interests and seemed to want to do the same things. They moved in together five years ago and even thought about adopting. But when Laura went back to college to retrain to be a teacher at the age of 34, Sally was not supportive. Laura made new friends and for the first time started seeing them independently. She eventually decided that she really needed to be independent for a while and moved out into her own apartment.

Relationships are defined by each partner bringing forth new things in the other. When this stops happening we are faced with several choices. We can go on as we are and feel more and more unhappy, we can talk about our problems and try to resolve them, or we can end the relationship.

From the mid-30s onward, dealing with relationship issues, psychological wounds, or emotional traumas from our past tends to take precedence. Prior to that, the business of living, establishing a career, having children, and so on, tends to obscure them. Younger women often feel too preoccupied to deal with all this what-is-the-meaning-of-my-life stuff.

The middle to late 30s continue to be a busy time. This is not to imply that being busy is the evil it is often made out to be. A study conducted by Wellesley College psychologists Grace Baruch and Rosalind Barnett in collaboration with Boston University journalism professor Caryl Rivers in 1983, known as the Lifeprints study, revealed how much has changed in women's lives in the past five decades. There was a time when women who worked felt alienated, but now it is those at home that often do. Those that had the greatest sense of well-being were, surprisingly, those women who seem the most likely candidates for burnout—those who were employed and married with children. The study proved that busy women often lead very rich and satisfying lives. The important issue here is whether a busy lifestyle is making you feel satisfied.

I have avoided the use of the phrase "balanced lifestyle" here because it is so often misinterpreted. As Borysenko rightly points out, there is a big difference between outer and inner balance. Outer balance is what we do with our day; inner balance is how we feel about it. Every day is a mixture of good and bad, and inner balance is what helps us cope with it. In our 30s perhaps our biggest challenge is living in the present and finally leaving the "I should be doing this or I should be doing that and what will other people think" mentality behind. If we can do that we are far more likely to feel satisfied with our lives.

Ideally, before we reach mid-life we will be well on the way to dis-covering what we want out of life. We will have learned that everything we have done in life, every experience, however dreadful, has some value. It will have helped us learn about human nature. And the wisdom gained from inner healing of old wounds, living in the here and now, balancing many different tasks, and doing what we want and not what others expect of us, prepares us well for the next phase—mid-life—when the wise woman in all of us can finally emerge.

Reaching 30 is a crisis point, but as Levinson, Borysenko, and Sheehy stress, life is a series of crises and turning points—some are just more marked than others. The 20s were all about experimenting, learning about ourselves. In our 30s we begin to question the choices we have made. To reassess our priorities. The crises we experience in our 30s are about searching for our true identity and becoming a adult. Like the odd wrinkle or gray hair, they are a part of the normal aging process. They propel us forward and help us grow and mature and truly learn about ourselves.

As time passes we mature and we learn, often through loss and disappointment, how important it is to constantly reassess our prior-ities, not just in our 30s, but throughout our lives. This is, of course, something we can only learn in retrospect with the wisdom that age brings, but hopefully it will ease some of the confusion about growing up and offer us some comfort.

Right now for those of us in the midst of thirtysomething angst we can't yet fully understand, the best way we can help ourselves is not by trying to intellectualize our struggles but by taking care of our health, both physical and emotional. Parts Two and Three show that understanding age-related bodily change in our 30s and paying atten-tion to our body's needs are ways we can become more supportive of our body and our life as it changes. They also stress that attending to our psychological and emotional needs is equally vital if we want to feel healthy and fulfilled as women.

PART TWO
AGE-RELATED CHANGES

"And so from hour to hour we ripe . . . "
—William Shakespeare, *As You Like It*

•   •   •

"You can't help getting older, but you don't have to get old."
—George Burns

Chapter 4
The Major
Organ Systems

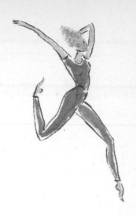

Like many women in their 30s, I found the changes in my physical body difficult to adjust to. It seemed so unfair that just as I was starting to appreciate what mother nature had blessed me with, age was starting to take it away. I was getting cellulite and tiny wrinkles. I wasn't truly young anymore.

If you, like me, are not prepared for age-related change, it can be an unpleasant shock when it does make its presence felt. It is hoped that the information given here about age-related change to expect in our 30s will ease some of the anxiety.

Most of us begin to notice the early signs of change in our 30s. We might wake up with aches and pains we never had before. We notice the first wrinkle. We can't lose weight so easily. Our skin feels dry, our hair is noticeably thinner. We haven't got as much energy. It takes longer to heal. We don't recover from colds so quickly. We look and feel older. Few of us are really aware, however, that all these visible signs of getting older are often the consequences of invisible changes that are taking place in our major organ systems.

There are several major organs in the body that are fundamental to life and which change over the years. These organ systems are the cardiovascular system, the nervous system of which the brain is a part, the immune system, the endocrine system, the reproductive system, and the skeletal system. All these systems are viewed as major sources of change in the body. Let's see what's happening to them in the 30s.

The Thirtysomething Heart

We know now that the cardiovascular system, although directly related to the leading cause of death in many countries, is not the cause of declining health. It is not your heart that deteriorates as you get older, but your arteries. The heart is tireless and would go on beating thousands and thousands of times a day for considerably longer if the system of arteries that supply it with blood were healthy. One of the main causes of poor health is narrowing of the arteries. Body tissues cannot be healthy if they do not get enough blood.

What has been discovered in autopsies done of male casualties of the Vietnam and Korean wars is that a large number of atherosclerotic changes begin as early as the 20s. Atherosclerosis, a thickening and hardening of the walls of the heart which restricts blood supply, is the leading cause of cardiovascular problems. It begins early in life and may later produce a heart attack, angina, or a stroke. So the relevant question in the 30s is not, "Am I likely to get heart disease?" or "Do I have it or not?," but "How much heart disease do I have?"

There is a glaring lack of information and advice for younger women about heart disease. Most women still live under the illusion that it is only a male disease. We worry much more about cervical or breast cancer than about heart disease, but heart attacks are the most common cause of death in women. They kill more women than men. Most of us would think that breast cancer would be the biggest threat to women, but without suggesting that breast cancer is not an important problem—it affects nearly one in nine women— heart disease kills five times as many women as breast cancer. Until recently, preventative research about heart disease was mainly concerned with men. This dreadful state of affairs is clearly the fault of the research system, which is now trying to rectify the situation.

Not only research, but public education for women about their hearts has been neglected. If women become more aware of what affects their cardiovascular health they can take steps to improve it.

Unfortunately, as long as so little is known about the nature of heart disease in women, doctors can only guess how best to prevent it. We can only follow the advice offered for men, even though the issues differ in certain important ways from those that concern men.

Although we tend to die of heart disease more than men, we do have an advantage. This advantage seems to be the protective effect of estrogen. On the other hand, certain hormonal disorders, when estrogen levels fall too low, can take away the normal female protection.

Risk Factors for Heart Disease

Many of us in our 30s don't consider ourselves at risk of heart disease. Not only might we think of it as a man's problem, but we also think that it is far more likely to occur after menopause. But women in their 30s have been known to have heart attacks, and these are much less likely to be accurately diagnosed and treated. What's more, the chances are that if heart disease does occur after menopause, arteries had already begun to narrow in the 30s. The way we lead our lives in the 30s lays the foundation for heart problems.

The only way to accurately assess this silent problem is to have a screening done while under a stress test like a treadmill. This test is worth paying for if there is a history of heart disease in your family. The National Cholesterol Education Program (NCEP) recommends that above-normal cholesterol levels be brought down considerably. Other doctors are not quite so enthusiastic, believing that cholesterol levels that are too low are unhealthy. They recommend only treating patients with very high levels and reassure healthy premenopausal women that they are not at risk. Despite differences of opinion, though, most doctors today do recommend that a woman has her cholesterol levels checked every five years from the age of 20. More frequent checks may be necessary if the following risk factors are present: if there is a family history of heart disease, if you are diabetic, if you smoke, if cholesterol is high, or if you suffer from hypertension. Having a parent, brother, or sister who has had a heart attack before the age of 60 is bad news whatever your gender.

Diabetes seems to be more ominous for women than for men. The U.S. Nurse's Health Study revealed that diabetic women had six times the risk of heart disease than nondiabetic women. This is because it is thought that the metabolic changes that accompany diabetes damage the small blood vessels supplying the heart. Other risk factors revealed by the study included high cholesterol, obesity, and high blood pressure.

Smoking is also thought to account for more than half of all premenopausal heart attacks, and it triples the risk of stroke before the age of 50. Smoking has an adverse affect on cholesterol and depletes free radical–attacking vitamin C. It also stimulates catecholamines, which causes arteries to restrict and blood pressure to rise. Many studies show that risk of heart attack falls rapidly when smoking is stopped. This has to be one of the most powerful arguments for stopping smoking before you reach menopause, when the risk of heart disease increases dramatically. So if you are in your 30s, if you smoke, and also take the contraceptive pill, which increases the risk of blood clotting, your risk of heart disease really takes off.

We know that cholesterol plays a role in the development of heart disease. Cholesterol is a soft, waxy substance that can be made in the body or ingested in food. Animal fat is the main source of dietary cholesterol. It is present in large amounts in eggs, meats, and dairy products. Cholesterol is a necessary substance for our bodies. It is essential for the formation of cell membranes and the actions of steroid hormones, which doctors think are antiaging. Why then is cholesterol always seen in such a negative light?

Before circulating in the blood stream, cholesterol must join with proteins to form particles called lipoproteins. There are high-density and low-density variants of lipoproteins. The low-density lipoproteins (LDL) are bad news. When an arterial wall is injured, LDLs tend to be deposited there. The repair process may end up producing scarring, which narrows the artery. The artery has no mechanism to remove the cholesterol, so what is deposited at injury sites tends to stay there. Over the years more and more cholesterol and scar tissue accumulates and the artery becomes narrower. Arteries are clogged and the risk of heart disease increases. High-density lipoproteins (HDL), on the other hand, are good news. They remove cholesterol from the arteries and return it to the liver for reprocessing.

If a woman has low levels of HDL and high levels of LDL, her risk of heart disease increases significantly. The trouble with cholesterol-lowering drugs is that they lower both HDL and LDL. While the debate still rages on about the wisdom of medication for poor cholesterol profiles, research has shown that HDL levels can be raised with diet and exercise. Exercise definitely raises HDL, and it does more in women with low HDLs than in those who already have favorable ones. However, several hours a week of aerobic exercise are required. Another way to raise HDL is to increase alcohol intake and enjoy a glass or two of wine a week. But there is no conclusive proof that alcohol-induced HDL is the protective kind, and alcohol has enough problems associated with it, so it is probably not the best way to correct your cholesterol profile.

There is much debate about how much cholesterol we should or should not eat and in what form it is best to eat it. Certainly avoiding saturated animal fats seems to be a way to lower cholesterol levels. Certain foods, like shellfish, have a high level of cholesterol, whereas other foods, like oily fish, have been shown to have lower levels. Having your cholesterol levels checked regularly by your doctor can detect any problems should they arise. Research shows that women with narrow arteries can actually unclog them to some extent when a sensible diet is followed. For once, things are a bit easier for us than for men. Male heart disease patients have to cut back to 10 percent total fat before such changes are seen, while women may be able to start clearing up their gummed-up arteries on about 20 to 25 percent total fat.

Hypertension, or high blood pressure, has been shown to increase the risk of heart disease. *The Silent Thief of Youth* is how it is described by the editors of *Prevention* magazine in *Age Erasers for Women* (p. 214). High blood pressure itself usually produces no symptoms, which may make it hard for you to believe you have a medical condition. Headaches can herald it, as can dizziness and ringing in the ears. Over years, however, high blood pressure can cause the heart to enlarge and eventually wear itself out, resulting in heart failure, a situation where the heart is no longer able to pump blood effectively. Because the arteries have to bear a pressure that is greater than normal they may burst, causing a hemorrhage stroke in the brain. Coronary heart disease may also result. Narrowing of the arteries that supply the heart occurs as a result of scarring due to vessel injury from excessive pressure.

Blood pressure normally gets higher as you get older and it would not be unusual to have the upper (diastolic figure) to be 100 plus your age, although the fitter you are the lower it will be. The bottom figure should never be higher than 90. If you are in your 30s you shouldn't worry unless your blood pressure is higher than 140 over 90.

Preventing and Treating Heart Disease

In your 30s it is wise to have your blood pressure checked every two years or so to see if it is within the normal range. If your blood pressure is very high there are medications to lower it. Regular cholesterol checks are also advisable. Women who are premenopausal and estrogen-deficient may benefit from estrogen therapy. Estrogen helps keep LDL levels low and HDL levels high. Aspirin also has positive protective effects against heart disease. This is due to the drug's effect on the smallest particles in the blood called platelets, which are instrumental in blood clotting. Aspirin can prevent blood clots from forming, not because it can stop the accumulation of fatty deposits in the artery, but because it can keep blood thin enough to keep flowing through. Aspirin, though, is not the right medication for everyone. It is important to consult with your doctor if you need medication for cardiovascular problems.

Medication for heart disease often has unpleasant side effects, and if at all possible it is better to treat the condition with lifestyle changes. And the sooner in life you act the better. Keep your weight down; most of us think of heart failure and being overweight as one and the same thing. Certainly too much body fat is a risk factor, but where that fat accumulates is a truer indicator of risk. If weight is carried around the waist there is a higher risk than if it is carried below the waist. So it's better to be pear shaped than apple shaped.

Certain experts believe that risk decreases if diet is improved. Smoking should be avoided at all costs. Other recommendations include cutting down on saturated fat, eating more fresh fruit and vegetables, and ensuring that you get enough of vitamins C and E, which seem to have protective effects and keep the blood vessels flexible and free from plaque that builds up and constricts the vessel, raising the pressure. Research is also making it clear that exercising regularly is important. Studies at the University of Pittsburgh have found that active women have lower blood pressure, lower total cholesterol, and higher HDL cholesterol than their sedentary peers, and suggest that regular exercise may protect against the increasing risk of heart disease. The heart responds to exercise. Recent studies have shown that negative changes in blood fat, which pave the way towards heart disease, start well before mid-life but they can be reversed by a regular program of exercise. Even walking is associated with big improvements in heart health.

One of the most frightening things about heart disease is that it can strike out of the blue. It is very difficult to screen properly for restrictive blood flow in the arteries. Rather like aging itself, the disease is an invisible process that slowly invades the body. But unlike aging, it is not inevitable; there are things you can do in your 30s to protect yourself against the very high risk of heart disease after menopause.

Over the last 25 years, as Americans have become more health conscious and taken action about their health, the death rate from heart disease has plunged. It would plunge even lower if more of us took action earlier in life. A heart-healthy lifestyle in the 30s is an investment for the future. So next time you find yourself munching your way through a packet of potato chips in front of the TV, think about what may be going on in those arteries of yours.

The Thirtysomething Brain

The nervous system controls your body's activities. Some researchers believe that the brain, which governs the central and peripheral nervous system, also governs age-related changes. For instance, the hypothalamus is believed to initiate the many changes associated with the female reproductive system, including menopause.

The phrase "There are three early signs of age: the first is loss of short-term memory and I don't remember the other two," is humorous because we have all been there. As we get older we do tend to get more forgetful. Our brains don't seem to function as well. We don't seem to remember as much as we used to. As the years pass we find ourselves writing more and more reminder notes.

The brain is an incredibly complex organ. It is composed of billions of nerve cells, or neurons, and supporting cells, all of which collect and receive information. Loss of brain cells occurs as the years pass by. One researcher calculated that in one part of the brain we lose an average of 100,000 neurons per day from the age of 30. That's 36,500,000 a year! Frightening, isn't it?

At age 30 brain weight is already beginning to decrease. At birth, the brain weighs about three quarters of a pound and increases to a maximum of three pounds around age 20. Brain weight then decreases, until at approximately age 90 it weighs about 10 percent less than it did at age 20. Loss in brain weight can be seen on the surface of the aging brain, where the grooves between the convolutions get wider. This change can now be visualized in a living person with a CAT scan. But before you panic, remember that exactly how the brain functions is still a mystery, that brain size does not indicate intelligence, and that recent research is reassuring us that brain neurons can and do regenerate.

While there is universal agreement that brain weight decreases, there is less agreement about what is lost, where loss occurs, and whether or not this affects our thinking skills. Cells and fluids are definitely lost and the brain changes *shape*, but where and how this happens and how it affects each individual is difficult to determine.

Brain deterioration has tremendous consequences for human life. Our ability to think and reason is what makes us human. Brain dysfunction tragically affects millions of Americans and destroys quality of life. Until about 20 years ago, it was assumed that "senility" was a natural part of getting old. But research inspired by Alzheimer, the German neurologist who in 1906 first described a form of cognitive impairment in humans, has increased public awareness. Alzheimer's is now considered a disease and not a natural part of age-related change. It is unpreventable and unstoppable and in time completely destroys thought and movement. It is believed that there is a gene responsible for the disorder and that those most at risk have several relatives with the disorder.

As well as Alzheimer's, vascular dementia and stroke can cause brain degeneration. Stroke happens when the brain gets blocked by blood clots. The result is a series of mini-strokes which can go unnoticed until a major stroke occurs. The number of women dying from strokes under the age of sixty is increasing, but most of these deaths could have been prevented by regular blood pressure checks, avoiding drinking and smoking, and treating diabetes.

Other factors affecting mental capacity include severe depression. Depression can, if left untreated, closely mimic Alzheimer's disease in the way it affects the brain. Medical conditions such as thyroid conditions and anemia can also limit mental capacity. Certain medications and drugs may too be responsible for diminished mental capacity. Even over-the-counter drugs for common ailments like diarrhea, nausea, and insomnia can cause memory loss.

Alzheimer's, strokes, and chronic depression are associated with getting older because they tend to strike in your later years, but it is important to point out that they are illnesses and not a natural part of the changes that come with age. We do not automatically get senile as we get older. Unfortunately, though, the idea that anyone approaching 40 is past their best mentally is an enduring one. It is responsible for a lot of age discrimination problems in our society. Some employers only hire the young, and some older people limit themselves because of their reluctance to start something new and their anxiety about the so-called first sign of old age: forgetting things.

Studies conducted in the 1920s that "proved" that intellect began to decline after the age of 20 continue to haunt us, even though these studies have long since been declared inaccurate and inappropriate. These studies, designed to predict academic achievement in children, did not take into account the fact that as we age our mental attributes develop and change. We can synthesize and integrate information better even though we may not have a gift for quick thinking anymore. Study the work of any great artist or writer, for instance, and you are likely to see some kind of a change in the mid-30s from inspiration that is spontaneous and rapid to more carefully crafted creativity. Look at Shakespeare's early tragedy *Romeo and Juliet* in comparison with his more mature *King Lear*. Both are equally superb, but in different ways.

We know that our brain does shrink gradually, that the number of neurons decreases, that the number of points of contact between cells decreases, that reaction time slows as blood flow decreases slightly, and that different parts of the brain alter at different rates, but the experience we have gained over the years in organizing material should make up for any loss of speed. Long-term memory loss is rarely affected. Skills we have learned will remain intact and may be so well ingrained that they become second nature. "To suppose that an individual peaks intellectually at age 20, and declines from then on, is to assume that intelligence owes everything to physiology, and nothing to accumulated effects of experience, knowledge, judgment and practice" (Hutton, p. 161).

Even though our brains do start shrinking in our 30s, a busy life with lots of distractions and lack of sleep is the most likely cause of memory loss. Many of us won't have the same powers of recollection we had in our 20s. But getting older is unlikely to be the real cause. In our 30s our lives tend to be far more complex than they were 10 years earlier. Before we know it our days are a list of things to do and diaries and organizers. With so much to do our minds often focus on the task ahead rather than the one in hand, leaving us dependent on list-making and memory jogs. We are not going senile; we just have much more to remember.

Many new moms joke that their brain shrunk when they had their baby, but this has more to do with fatigue and the distraction of looking after a demanding baby than anything else. Many women in their 30s, even those without babies, are chronically deprived of sleep. Surviving on a few hours of sleep because there is so much to do at work or at home will take its toll, not only on health, but on memory. Sleep specialists are coming to the conclusion that the lack of the right kind of deep sleep can make a woman underperform the next day. Sleeping pills aren't really the answer, because they don't produce the right kind of restorative sleep.

Memory loss that can't be explained by anything else probably won't become apparent until much later in life, but even then it won't be dramatic. The problem is that as we get older we get more sensitive about forgetting things. We make too much out of something very normal. Everybody forgets things from time to time. Occasional lapses of recall are natural at every age, particularly in this era of information technology and stress. Memory lapses also have a lot to do with the loss of vital nutrients to the brain because of an inadequate diet. Free radicals (discussed later) are notorious for causing memory problems, as are deficiencies of B vitamins.

So forget this myth of memory loss when you get past a certain age. If you feed the brain healthy food and keep using it those memory lapses that make you feel older than you are will be a thing of the past.

Keeping Mentally Fit

For those of us concerned about declining mental function, there is good news. The various vitamins, minerals, herbs, amino acids, and so on that claim to increase brain function are not as beneficial as the simple act of using your brain. Challenge, stimulation, learning something new, and staying current can keep mental deterioration at bay. Your mind does not have to disintegrate as you get older. Mental decline does not necessarily accompany graying hair and wrinkles. With motivation and commitment, you can be as sharp in your 70s as you have ever been. And if short-term memory isn't quite as good as it used to be 10 years ago, remember that getting older brings with it the rich compensation of wisdom and experience.

There is nothing that can make a woman look older than lack of mental challenge. In our 30s many of us will have settled down somewhat. Without knowing it, we can get stuck in a predictable routine. Without knowing it, we are prematurely aging. There is much truth in the saying, "You don't grow old, you only get old when you stop growing," and that means growing as a person. If you stop using your brain, stop learning, stop challenging yourself, and stop trying new things, you are old—whatever age you are.

The Thirtysomething Immune System

"I've been ill with the flu three times this year. I never used to get ill. I haven't moved to the city or anything, so why do I get colds so often?" (Nina, age 35)

The job of the immune system is to fight infection and illness. It is supposed to detect, inactivate, and remove microorganisms and other foreign materials from the body. "Proper performance is vital for survival" (Hayflick, p. 153). Immune functions do change as we get older, but how this happens varies from individual to individual.

The human immune system begins to develop just a few months after conception. It does not become armed to detect foreign bodies and produce antibodies until birth. By the time we reach our 30s, some of our cells will have incurred small changes. The problem is that the immune system is so sensitive that it will manufacture antibodies in reaction to these changed proteins. As a result the superb sensitivity of our immune system, which served us so well in our teens, may in fact cause us more harm than good in our 30s by attacking as foreign that which is our own.

Crucial to the performance of the immune system is the thymus gland. After puberty, for some mysterious reason the thymus degenerates, and it is believed that this triggers aging of the immune system. By the age of 50 we are only left with about 10 percent of the original mass of our thymus. Hormones released from the thymus begin to decrease around the age of 25. Certain white blood cells produced by the thymus, which are important for the proper functioning of the immune system, also decrease in number.

Once we reach 30, our bodies are less efficient at mounting an attack against illness. Not only is there a decline in the immune system's ability to produce antibodies, but there is also a greater chance that it will produce antibodies that attack harmless cells. The result is that not only are we more susceptible to illness in our 30s, but we take longer to recover. But declining immune system function in the 30s can be easily controlled. Making sure you lead a healthy lifestyle, getting all the nutrients you need, and reducing the amount of stress in your life are the best ways to boost your immune system and ward off illness.

The Thirtysomething Skeleton

Mandy is a recovering anorexic. During her teens and early 20s she severely restricted her diet. Finally she has managed to put her demons behind her, but her eating disorder has left a lasting legacy—weak bones.

Mandy is only 34 and she suffers from osteoporosis—a condition usually associated with older women. We have seen women who suffer severe cases. They are usually stooped, with eyes lowered to the floor. They walk very slowly and it is obvious that they often feel pain.

The idea that frailty and weak bones are part of getting old has contributed to the trivialization and neglect of osteoporosis. But for the last ten years increased public awareness of the condition has made it clear that osteoporosis can be prevented or at least diminished. We are also becoming aware that it doesn't only strike the elderly. Women in their 20s and 30s can suffer from osteoporosis.

Osteoporosis is a disease in which low bone mass and a deterioration of bone tissue lead to bone fragility. As a result the risk of bone fracture increases. Fractures and injuries can happen not just from a fall, but from simple everyday tasks such as bending and reaching. Fractures are most common in the bones that support the whole skeletal structure, such as the spine and hip bones. Wrist fractures are also quite common since the wrists can take the greatest impact from a fall.

It is believed that one in three women will at some point in her life suffer from osteoporosis. Genetics and race play a role here. The condition is most common among white, fair-haired women and Asian women, and is far less common among black women. Men also get osteoporosis but at a much lower rate. This is because men have much bigger skeletons and they don't suffer the effects of losing bone-friendly estrogen at menopause. Research indicates that bone loss is often due to estrogen deficiency.

The 206 bones in the skeleton are composed of compact bone, which is dense and makes up the bones' outer surface, and trabecular bone, which acts as a filler and is much lighter. It is trabecular bone that is vulnerable to osteoporosis. The skeleton is not, as many of us think, solid and unchangeable. Throughout our lives it is constantly being broken down and built up. The activity is ceaseless. Within bones there are living cells called osteoblasts, whose function is to make or form new bone. Other cells, called osteoclasts, break down old bone. This process of formation and absorption takes place throughout our lives, but in the very young, more new bone is made than destroyed. The bone density of young adults is continually increasing until peak bone density is achieved in the 20s. By the age of 30 we will have achieved peak bone mass, and after that a gradual decline will occur. This process is accelerated after menopause, when estrogen levels plummet.

Statistics associated with osteoporosis in younger women are not as well documented in post-menopausal women, but women in their 20s and 30s can lose up to 6 percent of their bone mass every year. Some specific factors predispose the condition. Early menopause, which is either surgical or natural, increases the risk of osteoporosis, as does a hysterectomy. Other causes of estrogen deficiency during the fertile years can also make bone problems more likely, such as irregular or absent periods. Problems with menstruation are common among young women dieting, dancers, models, and athletes. Treatment for certain conditions, such as Chrohn's disease, multiple sclerosis, and thyroid, liver and digestive problems, can also weaken bones. Poor diet, smoking, or putting your body under excessive stress due to overexercise or excessive dieting also increases risk. You could be vulnerable to broken bones, curvature of the spine, and joint deformities. If these are occurring in your teens and early 20s, bone mass is not developing at an age when bone formation should be occurring, and peak bone density may never be reached. The effects of this failure to develop skeletal strength may be devastating. An athlete, for instance, who has absent periods and a poor diet due to her training regimen could lose as much as 25 percent of her bone density. A bone fracture that is taking too long to heal, or was the result of a minor fall, or sudden back pain could all be warning signs.

In the years to come it is conceivable that cases of osteoporosis will rise even further as weight obsessed women who spent their teenage and early years starving themselves come of age and suffer the consequences of years of poor diet and estrogen-deficient menstrual cycles. X-rays of the spines of some anorexics in their 20s and 30s are now revealing the sort of spinal crush fractures that normally are seen in 70-year-old women.

As we get older our risk of developing osteoporosis increases because our skeletons begin to gradually lose their strength and resilience. The average white woman loses about a third of her bone mass in a lifetime. She may not feel the effects until she suddenly fractures a bone. From then on osteoporosis can devastate lives. It is a major cause of death and disability in women; it kills more than breast cancer, but not quite as many as heart disease.

Preventing Osteoporosis

"The scandal is that osteoporosis is largely a preventable catastrophe" (Hutton, p. 163). Like declining mental function, a frail skeleton is not a natural part of the maturing process. There is something you can do about it. Prevention should start as early as possible. Certainly by the time you reach 30 you should be doing all you can to keep your skeleton strong.

Research has shown that osteoporosis is largely preventable through exercise alone. Before the invention of labor-saving devices and automobiles, osteoporosis was only a risk factor for the wealthy and idle. The rest of the population had no choice but to walk and carry and bend and labor. All that exercise kept their bones strong.

Exercise, especially weight bearing exercise, is so important because it stresses the bones and encourages the skeleton to build more bone in response. Strength training also builds up muscles, which keeps the bones stable. And you don't have to exercise for hours every day to notice a difference. Almost any sort of exercise, even if it doesn't appear strenuous, is beneficial. Of course, the younger you start to incorporate more activity in your life, the better, but you can build bone mass through exercise at any age. It's important not to overdo the exercise though. Overtraining weakens bones.

Anything that strains the skeleton seems to be good for it. Surprisingly, carrying a little excess weight helps too. The more fat you have, the more estrogen you have to protect your bones. Carrying too much weight, though, often encourages inactivity. Pregnancy combines increased levels of estrogen and added weight, so women who have had children can be at less risk of developing osteoporosis.

Making sure your diet is rich in calcium and magnesium will also help prevent osteoporosis. Dairy products contain half of all dietary calcium and low-fat or skim milk has more of the mineral than whole milk, if you are worried about your weight. Try to avoid too much fiber and salt. Bran unites with calcium in the intestine and stops it from being absorbed by the body. More calcium-friendly forms of fiber are fruit, vegetables, beans, and lentils. Too much salt increases sodium levels, which are not calcium friendly.

Calcium needs magnesium to be incorporated into bones. If you don't get enough magnesium in your body to match the calcium intake, excess calcium collects in soft tissues and not bones, and causes calcium deposits and arthritis. Ensuring that you get enough magnesium, found in grains, vegetables, fruits, cereals, and almonds, is important. Vitamin D (eggs, milk, oily fish, cod liver oil, margarine) and vitamin K (broccoli, Brussels sprouts, green leafy vegetables) also play a part in bone health.

Calcium is important at any age, but especially at mid-life and during early adulthood, when bones are still forming. The National Osteoporosis foundation recommends an intake of 1,000 mg a day or 1,500 if you are estrogen-deficient. Some doctors think taking a supplement is better, because as we age we can't absorb calcium as well.

Preventative measures in your 30s should hopefully keep osteoporosis at bay, but at menopause, when estrogen levels drop, risk levels rise again. Hormone-replacement therapy, which restores a woman's estrogen levels to premenopausal levels, has been shown to halt or even reverse bone loss if it is taken for 5 to 10 years. However, not all women are comfortable with the idea of HRT, especially as osteoporosis does not develop in all postmenopausal women.

Bone-strengthening exercise and a calcium rich diet, and in severe cases estrogen-related therapy, are recommended for most of us in our 30s. Acting now could not only save your bones, but could possibly save your life too.

The Thirtysomething Endocrine System

"The endocrine system, which produces hormones that regulate the body's functions, has long been thought to play an essential role in producing normal age changes" (Hayflick, p. 155).

Hormones affect all the cells in the body, and our hormone levels are constantly fluctuating in our 30s. Hormones act by attaching themselves to a receptor on the cells they target, and research has shown that the number of these receptors also declines over the years. Some believe that changes that have been attributed to decreases in hormone production are perhaps due to decreases in the ability of target cells to respond to hormones.

The delicate balance of hormones in our bodies changes over the years. For example, weight gain, glucose intolerance, and diabetes are all related to the body's declining ability to maintain normal sugar levels. How the body uses glucose, a fundamental source of energy, is controlled by hormones such as insulin and glucagon, which are secreted by the pancreas, and growth and thyroid hormones.

In our 30s we are most prone to disorders of the hormonal system. These will be discussed in more detail later. According to endocrinologist James Douglas of the Plano Medical Center in Plano, Texas, it seems that in this decade mild imbalances barely noticed before begin to openly manifest. For example, the odd missed period becomes amenorrhea, when periods are absent for months at a time. Or facial hair growth dramatically increases and the odd pimple develops into full-blown acne.

As yet there is no conclusive proof that intervention with hormones can arrest or reverse age-related changes. Hormonal changes do seem to reduce the resilience of tissues and organs that in our 20s helped us react and cope with a number of stresses. Decreased ability to recover from burns or wounds, to cool down efficiently when we are hot, or warm up when we are cold, may be due to increased hormonal miscommunication. Menopause—an obviously normal age-related phenomenon—is triggered by changes in the endocrine system. Perimenopause and other problems with the reproductive cycle, irregular periods, infertility, PMS, and early menopause, which can occur in the 30s, are also hormone regulated.

Many experts believe that we can return balance to our hormonal system and fight aging through the food we eat. In *The Anti-Aging Zone* (1999), Barry Sears attempts to give "a practical insight into understanding how hormones control the aging process" and how lifestyle changes can alter that process. He offers convincing evidence that a hormone-regulating diet can be antiaging.

For more information about prevention and treatment of hormonal problems see Chapter 6.

The Thirtysomething Reproductive System

We are born with all the primary oocytes, cells with the potential to develop into eggs, that we will ever produce—about two million of them. But by the time puberty is reached we have lost about half of them. Very few of the eggs remaining at puberty go on to mature, escape from the ovary, and become expelled during menstruation. Fewer still get fertilized. At menopause the number of oocytes approaches zero and the reproductive cycle stops.

Oocytes age as we age. They are exposed to change from the moment we are born and are affected by our health, diet, and lifestyle. By the time we are in our mid-30s the odds of a harmful change having taken place have increased considerably. This is one reason that developmental abnormalities occur with increasing frequency in pregnancies of women in their mid-30s and older. Chromosomal defects are more common in the eggs of older women and account for a large proportion of the abnormal eggs produced by older women. There is decreased fertility and more likelihood of having a baby born with birth defects like Down's syndrome, which is known to be more common in babies of older moms.

I had my first baby when I was 33. I felt young but on my doctor's form I was described as an "aged mother." If I had been over 35 I would have been an "elderly primigravida." It took a while for it to sink in that, regardless of the fact that more and more women are postponing childbirth until their 30s, technically this is what I was—an aged mom. Even though sexual and emotional maturity often comes much later, biologically we are at our reproductive prime in our early 20s.

From the age of 30, circulating hormones for our reproductive system begin to decline gradually. There are gradual changes in the ovaries; and the weight and size of the uterus and vagina change, often becoming smaller. These changes may result in discomfort during intercourse. Breasts also begin to change in shape as hormone levels decrease, but how they change varies for each woman.

The Threat of Ovarian and Cervical Cancer

Ovarian cancer can strike women in their 30s, especially if there is a family history of ovarian cancer, if they have not had children, and if fertility drugs have been used. There are very few early warning signs and these are easy to miss. Abdominal distention and bloating, and frequent urination could all be attributed to other causes. Ovarian tumors are easy to miss, even with pelvic examinations. Because of this ovarian cancer kills twice as many women every year as cancer of the uterus and cervix, which are easier to detect. If the condition is picked up early enough the outlook is very good, but unfortunately it is often detected at too late a stage.

Screening for ovarian cancer is improving all the time, but there is still much progress to be made. Screening for another type of cancer that can affect the female reproductive organs, cervical cancer, is more efficient: the pap smear test. Unfortunately many women neglect to have this done regularly.

Pap smear tests are notorious for being inaccurate. Abnormalities are often missed and mistakes are made. Receiving notification that your pap smear yielded abnormal cells can be a terrifying ordeal.

For many of us in our 30s a negative result is our first encounter with our own mortality. We may feel perfectly well and the thought that there are dangerous changes and abnormalities taking place in the womb is disturbing. Frequently in a few months these abnormal cells rectify themselves and normality returns but there is always the fear that they won't. "I felt so fit and well," says Lindy, age 34. "That piece of paper from the lab changed how I thought about my body. I felt abnormal. I felt old. This was out of my control."

Fortunately, cervical cancer is within our control. If you have regular checks the likelihood of developing cancer is very small. Laser treatment for abnormal cells, should they occur, is safe and effective. The best way to protect yourself against both cervical and ovarian cancer is to stop smoking, as this can encourage abnormal cells to stay abnormal, and to get to know your body better. If there is anything abnormal such as pain or bloating, pain during intercourse, a change in bowel movements or non-menstrual bleeding, report it to your doctor.

In rare cases women in their 30s can suffer from prolapse of the womb—a problem usually associated with older women. In prolapses, the womb literally drops down and bulges out of the neck of the cervix, causing a lot of discomfort. It is often caused by very weak pelvic floor muscles, so the best way to prevent possible prolapse is to work on strengthening your pelvic floor. Squeeze and tighten your vulva several times daily, say when you brush your teeth or comb your hair. You could also see if you can stop a flow of urine mid-stream by powerfully contracting the pelvic floor muscles. Experts recommend that you don't do this too often, though, as you may risk getting an infection. There are other exercises you can do as well, like squats, which are also beneficial for the pelvic floor.

The Thirtysomething Metabolism

Because of the changing muscle-to-fat ratio, it gets harder and harder to stay the same size. Muscles require a lot of nourishment to do their functions and keep the metabolic rate high. Fat lowers the metabolic rate because it just sits there and burns calories very slowly.

Metabolism is the sum of all the numerous and complex chemical events that occur in our bodies. It is the fuel that runs our bodies, gives us energy from the food we eat, and helps us adapt to the environment we live in. The higher your metabolic rate, the faster you break down your food and the more likely you are to stay thin. Metabolic rate is determined by how much muscle mass you have. One of the major reasons your body shape changes in the 30s is the fact that your metabolism changes.

Studies have shown that as we get older metabolic rate begins to decrease. We don't break down food as quickly and tend to put on more weight. We don't adapt as well to environmental changes and the rigors of stress, flu, or travel become more difficult to tolerate.

George Backburn, M.D., associate professor of surgery at Harvard Medical School, told *Redbook* magazine that for most people metabolic rate is at its highest at age 27, then it starts slowing down by about 3 percent every five years. "Between ages 27 to 47, your metabolic rate could decline as much as 12 percent." In other words, if at age 27 you needed around 1,800 calories a day to function, you'll need only 1,692 calories at age 37. But if you continue to eat 1,800 calories daily, the extra 108 calories will translate into one extra pound of body fat every 33 days.

Metabolic rate slows down by a few percent every few years from the mid-20s as muscles gradually disappear. It drops even faster if activity levels drop too. Fat tends to accumulate more. The older we get the harder it is to shift weight. It makes sense to try and prevent fat from accumulating in the first place when we are in our 20s and our 30s.

The Thirtysomething Digestive Tract

"In my twenties I had a few friends in their early thirties. They really disgusted me when they started to talk about body functions all the time. Things like constipation and gas. It was embarrassing. I remember thinking *I'm never going to be like that,* and now look at me. I can't believe it, ever since I hit thirty these things have become interesting to me. I think it has a lot to do with the fact that I'm trying to take better care of myself now. How regular I am, how bloated I feel is important." (Nina, age 33)

For many of us, our stomachs get less tolerant over the years. Eating foods we are not accustomed to, stress, gallstones, eating too fast, eating on the run, irritable bowel syndrome, and food poisoning can all cause indigestion. It can also be caused by heart problems and stomach ulcers, so make sure you get yourself checked out if indigestion is persistent.

If you do suffer from indigestion, avoid fried food, spicy food, alcohol, caffeine, and eating too late at night. Stick to a healthy, fresh, high-fiber diet and try to eat slowly, thoroughly chewing your food in a calm frame of mind. Try also to avoid eating large amounts at one time. Smaller, more frequent snacks are easier for the digestive system to process.

Regurgitation or reflux is a common stomach complaint. As we age the esophagus, which keeps stomach acids inside the stomach, gets weaker and more uncoordinated. Smoking, carrying too much weight, lack of exercise and a poor diet can make it weaken sooner. You might sometimes feel a painful, burning sensation in your chest and throat as the stomach acid escapes.

There are many drugs on the market for reflux, and advertising companies, realizing just how common the complaint is, have stepped up the advertising campaign. Frequently we see a woman in her 30s, 40s, or older who wants to indulge in fatty food but fears the consequences. Someone takes pity on her and tells her about a tablet she can take before or after her meal which will stop reflux. We see her eating like a kid again with no adverse effects.

The problem with this kind of advertising is that it encourages the very behavior which is going to make reflux worse—indulging in food that isn't good for you. Rather than being reliant on a drug, it is far better to help yourself by eating sensibly, exercising, and watching your weight.

When we get older many of us become far more conscious of bowel regularity. There is still an obsession with regularity that lingers on from centuries ago when people blamed their ill-health on their bowels. All disease was attributed to fermentation and putrefaction in the bowels. Disease, even death itself, was seen as the result of a sort of toxic constipation. Even today the ideal of inner cleanliness is pervasive from regimented toilet training to laxative abuse and colonic irrigation.

Constipation does make you feel tired and heavy. It will give your complexion a dull glow. Contrary to popular belief, constipation is not more common in older women, but older women do tend to worry about it more. The bowels do not slow down with age. What slows down with age is our level of activity. Lack of physical movement can make the bowels sluggish. Some believe that anxiety and stress can lead to digestive problems and constipation. Activity stimulates the passage of food through the colon and eventually out of the body, keeping us feeling healthy.

Food, as well as exercise, will stimulate a bowel movement, especially high-fiber food early in the morning. Fiber is far more than bulk that helps sweep the food out of the system. It may also potentially offset some of the damaging effects of a high fat diet of refined food. Soluble fiber (fruits, vegetables, cereals, and oats) can lower the bad type of cholesterol and lower total fat absorption. Food that is fiberless will stay in the bowel a much longer time. Seventy-two hours or less is normal and less stressful to the gastrointestinal tract. In countries where people eat only unrefined foods, transit time of food through the intestinal tract may be as short as four or five hours.

When food lingers too long in the bowels, hardened feces may cling to the walls of the bowel, creating conditions that encourage the growth of harmful bacteria. There are some 400 types of bacteria in the bowel, and when the high-fat, low-fiber breakfast you ate on Thursday as you rushed to work isn't excreted until Monday morning, the balance of bacteria can tip in an unhealthy direction. The biggest danger, of course, is cancer. Colon cancer is encouraged by constipation and a sedentary lifestyle.

Protecting the health of our bowels is important in our 30s. Including sufficient fiber in the diet is essential. Fruit and vegetables are not only low in fat but also excellent sources of fiber. Eating less red meat and cooking meat lightly will also help. Eating breakfast will encourage regularity, as will plenty of exercise. Heading to the restroom when the urge strikes and not straining (since this can encourage hemorrhoids) are also important.

Hemorrhoids are varicose veins in the rectum that are caused by straining to pass stools. They are painful, itchy, and uncomfortable, and may affect your sex life. Trying to deal with them through improved diet, regular exercise, drinking more fluids, and not straining is probably the best course of action.

Watching the texture and consistency of your stools is another way to check for bowel health. The healthy stool was once thought to float while the unhealthy one just sat at the bottom of the bowl. Experts suggest today that the ideal stool is smooth, doesn't crack, and passes through without straining. Stools that are hard or cracked need more fiber. Bran will help, but too much can rob the body of bone-strengthening and (some say) colon-cancer-protecting calcium.

It really surprised me how many women I interviewed said that they rely on laxatives if they feel bloated. I myself have been known to resort to them for relief. Many women began to take laxatives in their teens and 20s, and the problem in the 30s is that the laxatives have less dramatic effects. The bowels are not completely emptied, and stronger laxatives are needed. If laxative use is excessive, this will upset the body's chemical balance and cause mineral deficiency. Even mild to moderate use of laxatives can cause problems and may even make constipation worse because the system gets lazy.

A few of the women I talked to spoke ecstatically about the wonders of colonic irrigation. Colonic irrigation involves pushing about 2 or more liters of warmish water up the colon through the anus using a clear plastic tube. Some nutritionists believe that this is taking the fear of constipation and unhealthy bacteria in the colon too far. Not only is it extremely uncomfortable but for those who have healthy bowel movements it is totally unnecessary. Also, the benefits of pushing upwards in the bowel when the usual movement is down is questionable. Other experts, however, recommend colonic irrigation on a regular basis to ensure healthy bowel function. This is probably one of those things you'll need to decide for yourself, and I encourage you to gather information to help you make an informed decision.

The Threat of Colon Cancer

Colon cancer, after lung and breast cancer, is one of the biggest causes of death among women. Most of these deaths could have been prevented by screening at an earlier stage. When the cancer has reached an acute stage and there is rectal bleeding, abdominal pain, and chronic constipation, it may be too late for treatment to be 100 percent successful. Early detection is crucial as colon cancer, like endometrial cancer, has a slow moving, premalignant stage in the forms of growths called polyps or adenomas.

When I was 32 I experienced anal bleeding. That and the fact that my mother had suffered from colon cancer encouraged me to go for a screening. I was examined with a sigmoidoscope. This is a instrument that covers the lower part of the colon to check for polyps and adenomas which could become the starting point for most forms of colon cancer. Removal of these growths could mean the difference between life and death in the years to come. Fortunately for me the doctor only discovered internal hemorrhoids.

Regular screening for colon cancer is on the increase as women become more aware of the potential risk. Polyps take between 2 to 19 years to become cancerous. Testing at any age after 30 would do no harm. Yearly tests to trace blood in the feces can also pick up colon cancer. Anyone with a family history of colon cancer should seek medical advice. Anyone who notices a marked change in bowel habit, pain in the stomach, bleeding from the rectum, and possible weight loss, must see a doctor immediately. Hopefully this is due to hemorrhoids or irritable bowel syndrome, but it is important to make sure.

If you do find blood on your stools or toilet paper, be concerned but don't panic too much. Rectal bleeding is common and may be due to tears or hemorrhoids. Blood that is not bright red but dark or mixed in with the stool or the passing of mucus deserves more serious attention. Fortunately for those of us in our 30s only a small percentage of colon cancers occur before the age of 50. But it is still worth checking out any pain, bleeding, and discomfort and also making sure that you get enough fiber in your diet, cut down on fat, and get sufficient exercise.

Irritable Bowel Syndrome

Another common complaint among the women I interviewed was irritable bowel syndrome. "My life was torn apart by irritable bowel syndrome five years ago. In my early thirties when I was working two jobs, going to college, and eating junk food every night my stomach would growl and I had terrible bouts of diarrhea," says Pippa, age 36.

Irritable bowel syndrome is a condition that is embarrassing and debilitating, and the symptoms include every bowel problem you could imagine: constipation, diarrhea, cramps, nausea, and bloating. Studies have shown that stress is a major cause. Eating meals on the run in a state of tension is a recipe for poor digestion. Calming down your life seems to be the best treatment for this condition. Eating your food slowly and carefully, monitoring foods that seem to trigger the problem, and watching your sugar intake are all ways to beat the problem. Massage can also really relieve bloating.

The Thirtysomething Bladder

Many women in their 30s notice that they have to go to the restroom much more often to empty their bladders. Moms especially may feel that pregnancy makes everything bigger except the bladder, which gets smaller!

Although many of us in our 30s are happy to discuss bodily functions like periods and constipation, we aren't so happy to discuss weak bladders or, worse still, incontinence.

Incontinence is associated with old age, but it shouldn't be. Studies have shown that women in their 30s and 40s regularly have bouts of incontinence. This incontinence ranges from a dribble when we cough or sneeze to complete emptying of the bladder if we can't find a restroom in time. Few of us would admit it, but it's likely that some of the sanitary towels we buy are for leaking urine to keep us dry. It may even be leaking urine that stops us exercising regularly.

The bladder is influenced by a set of muscles around the anus and vagina called the pelvic floor muscles, which support the bladder and uterus. When you squeeze these muscles the urethral sphincter shuts and urine stops escaping. They also tighten when there is sudden movement, like when you cough or laugh or make love, so that there is no leakage. If there is too much pressure and the muscles are weak, as they tend to be after childbirth, for example, urine is likely to rush out when sudden stress opens the bladder neck. This is called stress incontinence.

The pelvic floor muscles do respond to exercise. All of us, whatever our age and however strong we are, should exercise them as often as we can. Strong pelvic floor muscles keep incontinence at bay and also improve your sex life. About 50 or so years ago, Dr. Arnold Kegel developed an exercise to help women who were suffering from loss of bladder control. In the United States these exercises are known as Kegel exercises (more on them later).

Childbirth is often thought to be one of the major causes of stress incontinence. A lot, of course, depends on the type of labor and delivery and how much damage was done to the pelvic floor. Unless there were severe complications, normal bladder control should return in a matter of weeks if encouragement is given with strengthening pelvic floor exercises. Other causes of stress incontinence are obesity (the extra weight pushing down on the pelvic floor weakens it), constipation (especially if this is combined with straining), and frequent bladder infections. Weak abdominal muscles don't help either. Diabetes and smoking increase the risk of incontinence according to some studies. Once weakened, the pelvic floor muscles can be further weakened by very strenuous exercise, lifting, and carrying heavy things.

Incontinence is not a normal part of growing old, nor is it an inevitable part of childbearing. There is something that can be done about it. Severe cases may need more active treatment or surgery, but milder cases can be self-cured. Opinions vary on how this can be done. Going to the restroom every time we feel the urge to urinate is not recommended by some experts. Your bladder should be able to store about a pint of fluid. Going too often will mean that the urge to go comes on sooner and sooner. Urine held in the bladder does no harm—after all, that's what the bladder is for. When the bladder is almost full signals are sent to the brain to empty it but the urge to go can be easily postponed. Cutting down bathroom visits or time-tabling them, starting at one hour between visits and building up to three-hour periods, however, is considered unwise by other experts. Here the advice is to go as often as you can. Trying to stop your urine, it is argued, could result in the buildup of toxins in the urethra, which can cause infection, cystitis, or other problems.

Both schools of thought, however, do agree on other matters. Restricting excessive fluid intake, not drinking too much tea, coffee, alcohol, and soda, losing weight if necessary, and checking medication for side effects can all make frequency of urine less of a problem. Exercise is also crucial.

Kegel exercises for the pelvic floor muscles can in most cases control the problem. They are also advisable for all women in their 30s who don't have problems with stress incontinence. If you don't know where your pelvic floor muscles are, the next time you urinate hold the flow if you can. You can also place a few fingers into your vagina and squeeze tightly. The tighter your squeeze, the stronger they are. If you really can't locate them at all, make sure you ask an expert to help you. If you can locate them, Kegel exercises performed regularly will help you regain strength and tone.

Kegel exercises are simple, sharp contractions of the pelvic floor muscles. Initially start with short contractions and then build up to more sustained ones, holding for a count of five or ten and releasing gradually. As the muscles get stronger, start experimenting with positions. At first lying on your back with your buttocks raised, then lying flat, then sitting, then standing and even squatting. If you do this several times a day, in combination with regular abdominal exercises there should be a real difference in a month or so. Better tone probably won't cure stress incontinence entirely, but it will bring improvements.

The important thing is not to ignore the problem if you have it. And if you have noticed that you are urinating more often start thinking about your pelvic floor muscles. All thirtysomething women, whether suffering from bladder problems or not, would be advised to do their Kegels daily, to strengthen their abdominal muscles, and to avoid too much alcohol and caffeine.

Preventing bladder infections, like cystitis, which can cause pain and soreness, is also important. Try to drink six to eight glasses of water a day, urinate after sex to keep the vagina free of bacteria, and wear cotton underwear. If you suffer a bladder infection, drink cranberry juice, especially the unsweetened kind (sugar can weaken your bladder further). You may need to dilute it. For a few days after you contract an infection get plenty of rest and drink lots of liquids. This will allow your body to deal more effectively with the infection. Abstaining from sex is advised, as friction and foreign bacteria will worsen the infection. If you have regular infections, blood in your urine, and develop chills and back pains, see your doctor immediately.

The Thirtysomething Muscles and Joints

In my years as a fitness trainer, time and time again I would hear women in their 30s requesting an exercise program that wouldn't make them bulk up. They wanted to look light. I would see them pursuing with enthusiasm exercise programs which focused almost entirely on cardiovascular fitness. Jane, age 36, runs for about 45 minutes every day if she can. "I do it to keep the weight off mainly. I don't want to weight train 'cause I start looking really big when I use my muscles and I don't want that."

Jane is quite typical of many women in their 30s. "For all the lip service paid to a well-toned body, modern women are conditioned not to care too much for muscle, looking on it as yet more unfavorable flesh" (Hutton, p. 155). We worry so much about building up "ugly" muscles, especially in our legs. The ideal is long and slender, not short and strong. "I got so despondent," says Julie, aged 32. "I decided to run the marathon this year. I thought if the training for that didn't help me lose weight nothing would. I found that I actually began to gain weight. My trainer said it was because I was building more muscle in response to my training program. I was getting fitter. I realized then that fitness was not as important to me as looking slim and I dropped out of the training program."

Many of us in our 30s neglect to work on our muscle strength. The result is a progressive loss of muscle strength as the years go by. You may find it gets harder and harder to lift your shopping bags or your children or to climb the stairs or to walk quickly. All these activities are determined by how strong your muscles are. If there is little muscle strength, you may soon find yourself tiring in normal day-to-day activities. Far too many women are becoming unnecessarily feeble early in life.

Loss of muscle strength, like incontinence or osteoporosis, is not an inevitable part of getting older. How weak our muscles get depends entirely on how sedentary our life is and how we choose to use our muscles. Weakened muscles do not happen overnight. It is a gradual process. You don't suddenly wake up without the strength to squeeze a can opener. It takes years and years of lack of practice to get to that state.

Aerobic exercise will retain muscle strength, but most women in their 30s would be advised to also add some kind of strength training to their exercise program. Machines at the gym are usually best, but any activity that uses the body's large muscle groups will help. If you carry your groceries instead of having them pushed to the car, if you use the stairs instead of the elevator, you are keeping your muscles strong.

Women who do some form of strength training to build up muscle will decrease their risk of osteoporosis. Contrary to popular belief, you won't start looking heavy. It is possible to have defined muscles as well as a slim physique. And it won't take that much effort to get this muscle strength. Your ability to develop muscle mass as a 30-year-old is much the same as your ability when you were a 20-year-old. Just twice a week sessions of strength training will show increased muscle strength, improved bone metabolism, and elevation of metabolic rate. For a muscular but lean physique keep the weight low and increase the reps/set rather than increasing the weight.

Flexibility

As we get older, the ease of movement we so enjoyed in our youth can slip away quietly. The process is so subtle that only those of us very in tune with our bodies would notice it. Linda, age 30, is a professional dancer. "Oh yes," she says. "The thirties are more of a struggle than the twenties. Artistically I feel more expressive but physically I notice a big difference. It takes me much longer to warm up. I need to rest more and what I used to do with ease is now more of an effort."

Most of us aren't as body aware as Linda. We probably will take our mobility for granted until it threatens to desert us or we spend a day with our grandparents. "When I go out with my grandmom," says Rachel, who is 34, "I feel so lucky to have my good health. She has to concentrate on everything. Nothing is easy any more. Her frailty restricts her in everything."

Our mobility is one of the most important things in our lives. Rather than taking it for granted in our 30s, now is the time to preserve it by continually using it and putting our joints through their paces. Every time we use our joints there is an exchange of nutrients from the blood to the synovial fluid that encapsulates the cartilage around the joint. The cartilage must be kept awash with synovial fluid if it is not to dry out. It is inevitable that as we get older our joints get dryer but we can prevent them from drying out too soon. If the joints are not used and are deprived of blood and nutrients the cartilage gets worn, the bone thickens, and the joints become stiff and sore.

Women in their 30s do often complain of unexplained aches and pains, backache that lingers, and stiff joints. Most of these problems are simply caused by lack of movement in our sedentary culture. Since we sit around all day and shuffle instead of walking, our joints are never taken through the full range of movement.

It is important to make time to take your joints through the full range of movement—and this includes the joints of your spine. The spine is much more supple than many of us think. It needs to be moved and stretched every day. Long, slow stretches that are held for 30 seconds or so are most beneficial. Short, sharp, bouncy stretches are not. Think of your muscles and joints as pieces of elastic. Pulling sharply will tear the elastic. Gradually easing will gently stretch the elastic.

If you do notice your joints are stiffer than they were in your 20s, try to walk or swim more. A yoga or stretch class might be of benefit too. Yoga is designed to be of maximum benefit to your joints and to bring all of the actions performed by joints into play. You may think if you feel stiff that the last thing you want to do is move, but that is exactly what you should be doing. Warming up properly and then lightly exercising your joints is the best way to guard against future stiffness.

You will almost certainly feel older if you have a stiff, inflexible, aching back. Your back is your central support system. Lower back pain is widespread among women in their 30s. Sedentary lifestyles are often to blame. Even those who exercise regularly often spend the rest of their time at desks, or in cars. In fact, we spend so much time sitting down that our pelvises are beginning to resemble those of pregnant women.

Watching your posture and observing proper body mechanics when you sit, stand, and walk will help ease back pain, as will making sure that you don't sit or stand for long periods at a time. Back pain can be a symptom of a more serious condition so it is worth seeing your doctor, but in the majority of cases it can be prevented by improving your posture, learning how to bend correctly from the hip or squatting with a strong back, and by regular exercise. Strong stomach muscles will help, as will losing excess weight and avoiding sudden jerking movements. Put ice, rather than heat, on the sore spot. Bear in mind though that back pain can be caused by more serious problems, like fibroids in the uterus, so make sure you get yourself checked by a doctor if you suffer regularly from back pain.

Hopefully this chapter has shown you that with proper self-care and awareness you can prevent many of the health- or life-threatening problems associated with changes that occur in the major organ systems. Being in your 30s today means that you don't have to look forward to declining health, frailty, and loss of good looks. These are not inevitable parts of getting older. Many of the conditions once attributed to age-related change, like osteoporosis, have been shown to be preventable. Life after 30 is not a distressing journey to decrepitude. Many of our concerns are preventable with self-awareness and a lifestyle that doesn't overload our organ systems.

Now that we have seen what is going on inside your body, let's take a look at what's going on outside, the more visible signs of getting older in the 30s.

Chapter 5
Visible Changes in the 30s

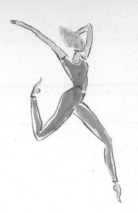

Knowing what is happening both inside and outside our bodies can help us accept changes in physical health and appearance that are inevitable, but at the same time enable us to prevent what is not inevitable. We've had a look at some of the systemic changes in the 30s and how they affect the entire body. Let's now consider the consequences of some of these aging events.

Your Height

"The normal erect posture characteristic of young adulthood is only rarely found in late old age" (Hayflick, p. 166). Our height doesn't usually begin to decrease until we are in our early 40s, but it can happen earlier. In our lifetime we lose about 2 inches in height with the greatest loss of height taking place in later decades.

Height diminution is thought to be due to a number of factors such as water loss, weakening of the muscle groups, postural changes, osteoporosis, spinal disk deterioration, and spinal deformities. In women, the predominant cause of decline in height is osteoporosis. As the last chapter showed, osteoporosis is preventable. And with proper attention to diet, exercise, strengthening muscles, and correcting posture we can do much to prevent height loss.

Your Shape

"I seem to be getting wider not wiser as I get older. It's harder for me to lose weight now. My body has made friends with my fat." (Sarah, age 31)

Putting on weight when you get older is a big fear for many women in their 30s. It's not hard to understand why. Our society is obsessed with youthful, perpetually adolescent standards of beauty. Being tall, firm-breasted, young, and thin, very thin, is today's cultural ideal of beauty.

The thin ideal has a powerful hold over women of all ages. Many of us object to it and can't live up to it, yet it lingers on. In the twentieth century, our ideal of beauty had changed dramatically, and then the standard of beauty has become increasingly more rigid and difficult to achieve.

Today plump is out and thin is in. We are pelted with messages telling us to be thinner, fitter, or more shapely. Next time you are in a bookstore take a look at the shelves of diet books and women's magazines that have the words "diet," "slim down," or "lose weight" on the cover. Small wonder that of all the effects of aging, weight gain is the one we worry about most. Small wonder that women are ten times more likely than men to have eating disorders, like anorexia or bulimia. In fact, eating disorders may just be the extreme of the universal spectrum. In today's culture, "to be a woman" writes Mary Pipher, "is to have a body image problem. For women harmful eating plans have become the norm" (*Hunger Pains*, p. 5).

Here are some alarming statistics gathered from women's magazines and news reports.

- Women overestimate their body size. We think we are fatter than we are.
- About 80 percent of us think we are overweight, when only about 25 percent of us are.
- Most of us hate our thighs, bottom, and stomach.

- The average American woman is 145 pounds and 5 feet 4 inches, but we wish we were 25 pounds lighter and a couple of inches taller.
- Every day millions of women in the United States are on a diet. The diet industry is booming.
- Many women don't want to stop smoking because they think it will make them put on weight. The birth control pill is rejected for the same reason.

A survey done among school girls in the 1990s reported that weight gain was feared more than nuclear war or cancer. If young girls are worrying about their weight at ever younger age, women are longing to be unrealistically slim at even older age. The desire to conform to the stereotypical thin image continues to exert its power as we age, even though it may have no relation at all to the age changes that take place in our bodies in the 30s.

Images of what the female body really looks like in the 30s are hardly seen anywhere. Those that are seen belong to women who have the figures of adolescents, which are more often than not obtained through years of dieting, exhaustive exercise programs, and maybe even surgery so that bodies conform to the young ideal.

Many of us in our 30s still have negative feelings about our bodies. We might become more reluctant to wear lycra outfits or strip down to a bikini on the beach. On the other hand, some women find that they become more comfortable with their bodies as they age. There is a newfound respect for the body and what it can do, perhaps brought on by childbirth or recovery from illness or injury when health was poor. Rather than starving and punishing themselves, these women prefer to be a little kinder to their bodies, taking better care of them through sensible diet, exercise, correct posture, and positive thinking. However we feel about our thirtysomething bodies, all of us have to come to terms with the reality that our bodies will change with age. That doesn't mean they will become unattractive. They will still be attractive, but in a different way.

Virtually every study shows that our weight increases as we edge towards mid-life and then decreases as we move towards old age. Weight gain tends to occur around the middle. In general, women in their 30s also have a chest diameter, circumference, and depth larger than they had in their 20s. There is also a gradual diminution in the length of the outstretched arm span. The thirtysomething face has nose and ears that have elongated with age, giving faces more definition as we lose the baby faced roundness of the 20s. The bones of the skull begin to thicken with age so that circumference, breadth, and length of the head increase. Rib bones continue to grow in the 30s and our palms also may widen gradually.

According to some studies internal organs shrink as we age but others show that some organs, like the heart, for example, get larger. There is general agreement that from the age of 30 the brain and kidneys begin to diminish in size. Skin folds increase and muscle mass decreases. For some unusual reason potassium levels also begin to fall slowly. Perhaps this is related to the replacement of muscle tissue over time with fat and connective tissue. Organ shrinkage could also be related to loss of body water. In our 30s just over 50 percent of our body is water. After mid life water drops to below 50 percent. This could be due to the actual loss of cells as we age or their reduced size. There is no evidence to suggest, however, that loss of water causes age changes.

Our bodies will change over the years. If you still weigh the same in your 30s as you did in your 20s your figure will have changed. It will be fuller in some places and more angular in others. Probably your tummy will be a little softer, your waist a bit thicker, your hip bones wider, your collar bones more pronounced, your breasts a little less high and full and maybe even the flesh on your arms a little less firm.

Generally you'll seem a little less firm because muscle starts to give way to fat in the 30s. How quickly this happens is, of course, very much dependent on you. Unless you work out religiously several times a week from the mid-20s onwards you will lose about half a pound of muscle for the same amount of fat every year. The consequence of this is a spreading middle, bottom, thighs, and clothes that seem to have shrunk in the wash. Since fat weighs less than muscle you may be delighted to see that you have lost a bit of weight but depressed to discover that you have gone up a dress size.

Body Fat

A body fat percentage between 18 and 24 percent is the ideal, but it is important to keep a sense of perspective. Even though your shape may change somewhat and you may worry that your waist is thicker you could still be well within the recommended range. In fact, the results of several studies on stored fat have found that in the middle years a modest increase in fat mass over what is considered ideal in the height-weight charts favors increased longevity.

If you look at the BMI chart (Figure 1) you can see that although a BMI between 19 and 21 may be preferred for appearance's sake, from a health point of view you are just as well off with a BMI of 24 or 25. Obviously obesity is a severe health risk, but all in all you can afford to gain a few pounds in your 30s. Weight gain with age may even be necessary—it may be mother nature's way of giving us more fat when we eventually stop producing estrogen at menopause. Expect to be a few pounds heavier in your 30s than you were in your 20s. In some cases trying to stay the same weight may not always make us look younger but give us a gaunt and haggard look.

A few extra pounds in the 30s won't make you look older but if weight gain is excessive it will certainly age you. Too much weight is a health risk. Recent research is indicating that straying more than five pounds over your ideal weight can accelerate the aging process. Be especially concerned if too much weight gathers around your waist. This is associated with increased risk of ill health. Often referred to as male-pattern weight gain, the pot-bellied apple shape, with a poorly defined waist, is associated with diabetes, heart disease, and maybe even infertility and cancer. As hard as it is to believe, the familiar

Figure 1

BMI (body mass index) Rating

Height	Your BMI	19	20	21	22	23	24	25	26	27	28	29	30	31
		Optimal Weight						Weight				Overweight		
4' 10"		91	96	100	105	110	115	119	124	129	134	138	143	148
4' 11"		94	99	104	109	114	119	124	128	133	138	142	148	153
5'		97	102	107	112	118	123	128	133	138	143	148	153	158
5' 1"		100	106	111	116	122	127	132	137	143	148	153	158	164
5' 2"		104	109	115	120	126	131	136	142	147	153	158	164	169
5' 3"		107	113	118	124	130	135	141	146	152	158	163	169	175
5' 4"		110	116	122	128	134	140	145	151	157	163	169	174	180
5' 5"		114	120	126	132	138	144	150	156	162	168	174	180	186
5' 6"		118	124	130	136	142	148	155	161	167	173	179	186	192
5' 7"		121	127	134	140	146	153	159	166	172	178	185	191	198
5' 8"		125	131	138	144	151	158	164	171	177	184	190	197	203
5' 9"		128	135	142	149	155	162	169	176	182	189	196	203	209
5' 10"		132	139	146	153	160	167	174	181	188	195	202	209	216
5' 11"		136	143	150	157	165	172	179	186	193	200	208	215	222
6'		140	147	154	162	169	177	184	191	199	206	213	221	228

female pear shape (heavy around the bottom and thighs) is good news. The chart given (Figure 2) will help you assess your waist to hip ratio to see if you are in the risk area. If you are, don't despair, weight around the waist is far easier to shift than weight in the hips. It is sensible in your 30s to start regularly checking your waist to hip ratio because hormonal changes over the years can affect where fat accumulates in your body.

Figure 2

Waist to Hip Ratio Chart (for women)	
Waist to Hip Ratio	Risk Level
1.1	very high risk
1	very high risk
0.9	high risk
0.8	high risk
0.7	low risk
0.6	low risk

WAIST TO HIP RATIO: Measure your waist and hips at the widest point and divide the first by the second. Check the results against the chart.

Heart disease, cancer, and diabetes are all associated with weight gain, but these do not become serious threats until BMI reaches more than 30, when weight should definitely be shifted for the interests of health. Lesser degrees of weight gain are not life threatening. In fact, some studies have shown that being slightly overweight increases survival rates. For most of us, then, the problem is not concern about our health, but concern about our appearance.

Just because you have always been a size 6, 8, or 10 does not mean that you must continue to stay that size in your 30s. Part Three will give information about weight loss and weight loss plateaus but if you are eating sensibly, exercising, and just a few pounds over your target weight you have to think about whether you have reached a weight loss plateau or not. Are you really overweight or is it time to consider accepting your natural weight? Remember, there is no law that states you must stay the same clothing size all your life, and being thin does not always mean looking attractive.

"I once used to train a client," says Susan, age 38. "She wanted a 6:00 A.M. aerobic workout five times a week. She was thirty-six and as thin as a rake. She smoked to keep her weight down and was obsessive about maintaining a weight of 110 pounds for her five-foot-five frame. I tried to tell her that she would actually look better a few pounds heavier but she wouldn't listen."

When we were 16 we could look good at a ridiculously low weight. In our 30s if we get too thin we start to look skeletal. Watch Hollywood movie stars when they hit their 30s. Being extremely thin doesn't always make them look younger. In fact it can make them look gaunt. Being superslim does not always mean you will look more attractive. This is especially so if severe dieting has taken place.

Drastic efforts to keep weight down in the 30s can ravage looks. Crash diets draw on ever decreasing muscle reserves or succulent fat just beneath the skin. Older skin doesn't ever contract back to its old shape as well and crash diets and too-rapid weight loss can give you wrinkles and saggy skin that won't go away. It is important that weight loss is gradual because once skin has stretched it won't shrink back to its normal shape. If weight is kept within the normal range in your 30s this may never be a problem. You won't need to opt for plastic surgery.

Bulges unresponsive to diet or exercise can be dealt with by suctioning out with liposuction or cutting it out with the surgeon's knife, but this is a drastic step to take that can be avoided if permanent changes in diet and lifestyle are made at a young enough age. And from the interviews I conducted with women who as a last resort decided to have liposuction, I learned that it is not the easy, inconsequential operation many of us may think it is. It is uncomfortable, often painful, expensive, time consuming, and may leave you with big scars, large bills to pay, and a long convalescence.

Why You Shouldn't Diet

Dieting can give you a burst of energy but, more often than not, it can be aging and frustrating. Time and time again studies have shown that diets don't work. As soon as the diet is abandoned, weight piles on again.

Keeping weight within the normal range should never be achieved with drastic dieting or yo-yo dieting. Constantly losing weight and then immediately regaining it is bad for your health. Dieting for weight loss and counting calories will also probably not work in the long term. You may find that there is initial weight loss, but time and time again weight is regained. This is because the minute you begin a restrictive diet your body translates this as starvation mode. It lowers its metabolic rate and breaks down food much slower. Basically your body adapts and is able to survive on less. The result is that you don't lose weight even though you are eating less and probably not getting the right nutrients for your body to function optimally.

Fluctuating in weight puts a huge strain on your heart and also your skin, which loses tone after all the times it has stretched and then been expected to bounce back. According to Gerald Imber, a leading cosmetic surgeon, "losing and gaining weight is one of the most aging things you can do" (Spillane and McKee, p. 152). Studies back him up. Rapid weight changes not only decrease your life span, they also make you look older. Better to keep those few extra pounds than to keep losing them and gaining them back again.

Dieting shrinks the body's muscle stores and drives down its metabolic rate. Calorie counting is even worse because no two calories are the same. You can eat 1,500 calories worth of chocolate a day or 1,500 worth of fruit and vegetables. Although both supply you with calories, the former won't give you the energy to function optimally and in fact will result in severe nutritional deficiency if continued.

If you want to lose weight the only really effective way is to change your eating patterns for life and increase your activity levels. Studies have shown that those who exercise regularly put on less weight as they age than those who don't. Regular exercise will trim the waistline and encourage a healthy muscle-to-fat ratio. Your belly may still be softer and your hips rounder and your weight may not change that much, but you will raise your metabolic rate and keep weight gain under control.

You need to make sure that you are getting healthy, fresh food that contains all the nutrients your body needs and which gives you enough energy to function optimally, Part Three will lay down guidelines for a healthy diet, which in combination with regular exercise, can not only keep the weight off but keep you looking and feeling young.

Your Breasts

Your breasts won't look the same in your 30s as they did in your 20s. They will change both in appearance and in composition. Childbirth and breastfeeding will certainly alter how they look. How a bustline changes with childbirth varies from individual to individual, but many moms say that their breasts were never quite the same after their baby. Many say that they look smaller and are more tear shaped rather than round and high.

But it is not only motherhood that changes your bust. Other factors are at play. From our early 30s onward hormonal changes that lead up to menopause begin to replace glandular tissue with fat. This, in combination with the downward pull of gravity, results in breasts that look flatter and are less firm, and nipples that seem to be looking at the floor.

This is not to say that women in their 30s have unattractive breasts. Quite the contrary. They are neither better nor worse than they were ten years ago, just different. The problem is not necessarily appearance but how changes in the breasts affect your self-esteem.

Breast Cancer

Just six months after I had my baby my doctor found a lump in my breast during a routine checkup. I was told to schedule a mammogram. I had to wait a week until my appointment and that week was an ordeal. It was hard to focus on anything. The thought of breast cancer was terrifying. Thankfully, my scan revealed nothing malignant, just a blocked milk duct, but that week of fear and the anxious five minute wait for my mammogram results were experiences I don't want to repeat.

We all live in dread of finding a lump in our breast, and as we age this fear intensifies. Breast cancer is not the most likely cause of death for women (heart disease is) but it is fast becoming a great threat to our health.

Doctors and researchers don't really know what causes breast cancer and why we are at greater risk the older we get. The number of new cases diagnosed per 100,000 cases rises drastically depending on the age group. Having a family history of breast cancer is thought to be a risk factor, as is having children at a later age, but some women who develop breast cancer don't have any of these so-called risk factors at all. There is cause for concern if your mother or sister had breast cancer before the age of 45, but if it developed after the age of 55 or if your aunt, grandmother, or cousin got the disease, your risk factor is only minimally raised.

Most of the changes in the breast that occur from our mid-30s onward are found to be harmless. A small minority, however, are not, and the risk of breast cancer increases.

It is believed that breast cancer is directly connected to estrogen levels. If menarche was early and menopause was late a woman has been exposed to great amounts of the female hormone, and the risk of breast cancer increases. This is because estrogen is a growth-promoting hormone that stimulates cell division. With each division the chance of a cancerous change rises, and when a tumor is present it may start to depend on estrogen for survival. Not having children or having them late in life is also thought to increase the risk of getting breast cancer. Breastfeeding for several months seems to have a protective effect according to some studies.

Estrogen levels are also raised by certain fat cells in the body. It is thought that fat stored around the waist increases risk far more than fat stored around the bottom and thighs. It is also thought that alcohol helps convert the hormone androgen into estradiol, a form of estrogen, so even though a few glasses of wine may reduce the risk of heart attack, they may increase the risk of breast cancer.

Research has also discovered that a country's rate of development of breast cancer seems to correlate with a high fat diet. Japanese women, for instance, suffer far less from breast cancer than American women. This is because higher than normal levels of fat in the body provide the conditions in which abnormal cells prosper. However, recent studies have also been showing that too much has maybe been made of the link between breast cancer and fat. On the whole, doctors recommend that women lower their fat intake on the grounds that it may protect them from breast cancer as well as keeping their weight down, and decreasing the risk of diabetes, blood pressure, heart disease, and colon cancer.

Studies have also shown that certain foods seem to have a protective effect against breast cancer. They include fruits and vegetables together with natural forms of vitamin E, such as tuna in oil, nuts, avocado, blackberries, and beta carotene–rich foods, like broccoli, carrots, orange/yellow fruits, spinach, soy, and Brussels sprouts.

There is no real evidence that a low-fat diet and avoidance of alcohol are protective against breast cancer, but the strong association with decreased risk should be enough to prompt many of us to consider changes in lifestyle and diet. Unfortunately, making changes in the 30s, although extremely beneficial, may be just a little too late. Recent research is showing that the vital period is in adolescence, when breast tissue is forming and at its most sensitive. It seems that exposure to the pill, alcohol, and a diet high in fat, is most significant in our teens.

Prevention

So what is the best way to help ourselves in the 30s? Experts agree that the answer lies in breast awareness. Get to know how your breasts feel. Breast self-examination is wise, but don't let it lull you into a false sense of security. Many of us are not trained to detect minute changes that perhaps only a mammogram will expose. It is important that all women in their 30s go in for yearly checkups.

Doctors are more likely to detect problems than we are, but being aware of how your breasts feel is a plus. The best way to check for any changes is to stand before a mirror and tense your chest muscles to check for any skin changes or changes in your nipples. Raise your arms and turn from side to side. Using a soapy hand, use the flat of your middle three fingers to make small circles from the armpit in toward the center to feel for unusual lumps or changes. Look for something that feels different from the usual lumpy texture, something the size of a small marble. Keep your movements light. You can miss small lumps under the skin if you press too hard. If you find yourself feeling uncomfortable with this technique, ask your doctor to do it for you.

Over the age of 50, twice yearly mammograms can catch signs of breast cancer early. It is a different story for the under 50 age group, though. The benefit of regular screening for younger women is still thought to be small. There is, in fact, little justification for low risk women in their 30s to have mammograms. In your 30s your breasts are often too dense in tissue for mammogram readings to be reliable. However, it is still vital that you are aware of how your breasts feel and that you ask your doctor for regular checkups and get a mammogram if there is any cause for concern.

If you are at risk, say a first degree relative had premenopausal breast cancer, or you have a condition that predisposes you to breast cancer, a regular yearly mammogram is perhaps the best way to detect early signs. X-rays are controversial but as far as breast cancer is concerned they can reveal far more than any doctor can with an examination. By the time you can feel a small lump in your breast it is already several years old and mammograms can bring the problem to light years before they are felt. Surgery can remove the lump and surrounding tissue and with luck it will not have spread to other cells in the body. If the cancer is found early enough before it spreads to the lymph nodes, the survival rate increases tenfold. Some experts argue that there is no way of knowing whether it would have ever developed into full-blown breast cancer. But waiting around to find out is something very few women would feel comfortable with.

Should problems be detected, modern medicine has now reached a point when surgery often spares the breast as well as your life. If the tumor is small the breast will soon regain its former shape. If a full mastectomy is advised, it is important to always get a second opinion.

With advances in modern medicine, blood tests may be able to identify women at high risk and safe drugs may be developed to reduce the recurrence of the disease. Until then, however, we have to rely on what we know and start getting into the habit of breast awareness in our 30s, if not before.

Your Thirtysomething Skin

The skin is the largest organ in the body. It consists of a thin outer layer, the epidermis, and a thicker layer underneath, the dermis, where the hair, sweat glands, and sebaceous glands originate. Collagen is present in this layer. The epidermis is strong and includes an outer layer of dead cells, which must be removed regularly. The dermis contains nerves, blood vessels, and living cells. As we age, cell renewal slows down from around 28 days to 40, and the epidermis and dermis appear to get thinner.

The skin is an incredible organ. It not only holds us together, but it can also breathe. It inhales oxygen and expels body toxins. It is only via the skin that we can absorb vitamin D from the sun and prevent bacteria from entering our system.

Skin shows dramatic changes as you get older. You can demonstrate the reduced suppleness and loss of elasticity as you age by pinching the skin on the back of your hand. Under the age of 40 it shouldn't take more than a second or two to snap back to its former shape. In your 70s it could take up to a minute.

Nothing determines our stereotyped opinion of a woman's age more than the appearance of her skin. Its discoloration, wrinkled state, and deterioration are commonly regarded as a reflection of chronological age, and even of general health. Other than what we are wearing, skin is what we see when we look at each other. Small wonder that aging is first recognized in the skin.

Deterioration begins in the 20s when the skin starts slowing down rapid cell regeneration and natural oil protection, but the changes aren't usually noticeable until the 30s, when many of us notice the first wrinkle.

Wrinkles

"The first time I saw definite wrinkles around my eyes I freaked out. I was getting old." (Lara, age 37)

The true blame for the anxiety many women feel at the sight of the first wrinkle lies not with the wrinkles themselves but with society's devaluation of older women. Eventually all of us will come to a more sensible response to the change, but the first signs of wrinkles in our thirtysomething years can have profound psychological effects.

Fifty years ago women didn't start to wrinkle until much later. In their 30s the wrinkles caused by natural aging were largely absent. "Doctors say that the inevitable wrinkles from genetics and gravity really shouldn't arrive until you near your sixties. But they come a lot earlier in the late twenties or early thirties—for many of us" (*Prevention* editors, p. 385). Why are so many of us noticing changes in our 30s?

There are many causes, but the principal one is the sun and the modern love of tanning. With few exceptions, early onset wrinkling and skin lesions are not the result of normal aging but represent the accumulation of environmental assaults. The main cause of the skin changes we see is the ultraviolet component of sunlight, which produces an effect called photoaging. The effect is greatest on skin exposed to the sun and least common on unexposed areas like the buttocks. If you are or have been a sun worshipper you will pay the price with deeper and earlier wrinkling. This is why dermatologists recommend that everyone, regardless of how naturally dark their skin may be, use high-protection sunscreens every day, even in winter. Sunscreens can also prevent the occurrence of skin cancer and its most dangerous manifestation, melanoma.

One of the major causes of premature aging is regular overexposure to the sun. In our 20s we could tolerate long spells in the sun but we can't do that in our 30s without getting wrinkles and dry skin. The ozone layer that protects us for the harmful rays of the sun has been getting thinner and thinner. In some parts of the world there are even holes in the ozone layer, which means that without protection you could literally burn up. This is not intended to destroy your enjoyment of the outdoors. It is well known that sunshine boosts our moods and supplies us with much needed vitamin D. But we all know the difference between a walk in the sunshine when the sun isn't too strong and lying in the sun for hours in the middle of the summer.

Smoking is the second major cause of wrinkles. The number of women smoking in their reproductive years has risen dramatically over the decades. Smoking reduces blood flow to the skin so that cells can't repair themselves. It also causes lip creases and creases around the eyes because of both the constant sucking motion and wrinkling of the eyes.

Sun, smoking, and exposure to environmental toxins are the principal reasons why many of us are getting wrinkles earlier than our mothers did. It is thought that the characteristic wrinkles that we all get with age are due to losses of a protein called collagen. Collagen is abundant in the body. In the skin collagen supplies stretchability, allowing the skin to expand as in pregnancy and then return to previous shape. In young skin that has not been overexposed to the sun, collagen fibers crisscross in an orderly fashion. But as the skin suffers sun damage these neat orderly bundles become disrupted and the individual fibers weaken. An enzyme called collagenase, normally used to destroy old collagen, starts to create inelastic tissue. This process is what makes sun-ravaged skin look so terrible. Natural wear and tear could never create the same kind of damage.

Yo-yo fluctuations in weight can also accelerate the aging of skin that no longer has the elasticity of youth. Stretch and sag marks are left, which no amount of exercise and diet can take away.

Some wrinkling is also related to muscle use. Habitual smiling and frowning will accentuate the formation of wrinkles at right angles to the pull of the muscles used. This may explain wrinkles around the forehead, mouth, and corners of the eye. The skin on the lips and eyes is the thinnest and most vulnerable, and the first signs of aging appear here. This is why eyes and lips require special care in the 30s. Other muscles in the face, chin, and neck are thought to cause wrinkles that parallel the direction of the muscle pulls in those area. Other wrinkles are not related to muscle use. Ear lobes, for example. Why do our ears enlarge and develop wrinkles with age? It is possible that ear lobe wrinkles, as well as irregular or crisscross wrinkles on the face, where facial muscles do not seem to play a role, may result from underlying changes in fat and connective tissue.

Dry skin can be caused by too much ultraviolet radiation.

Regular use of sunscreen will provide protection and keep the skin's own moisturizing ability intact. Harsh chemicals and excessive use of makeup can also dry out the skin. Many dermatologists rate humidifiers above day and night creams in keeping skin moisturized. Humidifiers hold upward of 40 percent of water in the atmosphere, a boon in heated and air-conditioned houses and work environments where humidity is often kept low for electronic equipment.

Alongside wrinkles, a few of us in our 30s may notice age spots cropping up. Also known as love spots, these are brown spots that can appear anywhere on our skin. Most often you'd find them on the hands but they are also common on the chest, neck, face, and other areas exposed to the sun regularly.

The skin is prone to pigment changes, and age spots are part of the natural aging process. Watch out for skin cancers, though, which need urgent medical attention. It is possible to camouflage age spots with cosmetics, but the best way to avoid them is to use your sunscreen and practice good skin care. For some reason, once you have age spots cold weather seems to make them worse.

Rosacea is an embarrassing skin condition that rarely flares up in the 30s, but if it does it gives the appearance of a permanent blush with swelling, dilated blood vessels, and sometimes pustules. There is not much that can be done about it so prevention is the best cure. Exposure to too much heat for too long a time is thought to be a possible cause. Try also to avoid hot and spicy food and extremes of hot or cold temperature.

Warts and other growths are also a natural part of getting older. In our 30s we are unlikely to notice them yet. Should you get warts you just have to live with them unless they make you so unhappy you want medical help to remove them. However, any growth that is darker than skin color, that bleeds, or that has a discharge, requires urgent medical treatment.

Many women in their 30s may also notice that all of a sudden they get hair in places they don't want hair. Mustaches, beards, and sideburns threaten to appear unless there is a religious approach to plucking. Whiskers that appear in the 30s are often the result of an underlying hormonal imbalance when there is too much male hormone circulating. This condition is known as an androgen disorder and will be dealt with more thoroughly in the next chapter. Unwanted hair can be removed by razors, tweezers, electrolysis, and creams.

Cellulite

Helen, age 34, is frantically trying to get rid of her cellulite. "I've lost weight. I would feel good about myself but I can't—I've got cellulite. Whatever I do it won't go away. It's not fair."

Cellulite. We all know what it is. Lumps of cottage-cheesy-looking skin that can hang on our thighs giving them an orange peel appearance. However much we diet and exercise they won't go away. Rare in our 20s, in our 30s cellulite is a big concern for many of us. Even the late princess Diana was upset when the British tabloid press accused her of having cellulite. Our thighs don't look and feel young anymore. Worse still, cellulite tends to increase with age. Cellulite is not life threatening, but from the way many women react to it you would think it is.

There are many theories about what causes cellulite. Why some women get it and why some don't. Stacks of books and magazine articles are devoted to it. Some believe that it has to do with poor circulation and poor lymphatic drainage. Others say that it is the result of malnutrition and stress and too much coffee, alcohol, cigarettes, and sweets. Others think that women with cellulite often have low esteem. Others that it is genetic. So far, no product on the market has effectively proved that it can banish cellulite. The creator of the one that does will no doubt become a billionaire overnight. Until then, if cellulite has not yet reared its ugly head, regular exercise to improve circulation and a healthy diet seem to be the best means of prevention. That as well as good genes, as cellulite is often inherited, and a large dose of good luck.

Other Skin-Related Age Changes

Levels of the hormone androgen control many of the sweat glands, and from the mid-30s androgen levels begin to decline gradually. Probably you have not noticed it yet in your 30s, but as you approach mid-life you may well find that you sweat less and have less need for deodorant.

The body's temperature control also becomes a little less efficient. The density of the skin's blood circulating system, consisting of small veins, capillaries, and arterioles is reduced with age. You may find it harder to warm up or cool down.

You could also find that your skin is less sensitive to pain. Injections don't seem to hurt so much anymore. This is because as we get older the nerve cells in the skin get less efficient with age and we feel less pain. This less efficient nerve response coupled with a decline in the immune system may also account for a reduced or slower inflammatory response to irritants. It may take longer for wounds to heal, for example.

Your Vulva, Vagina, and Cervix

The vulva and the vagina form the outermost points of entry into the female genital system. The cervix and its opening form the entryway into the uterus and inner pelvic organs—the tubes and ovaries. Changes in your vulva, vagina and cervix in your 30s very much depend on whether or not you have had children. A doctor can tell whether or not a patient has ever borne children just by looking at the opening of her uterus (cervix). The cervix of a woman who has not had a child is very tiny; generally that of a mother is larger and irregularly shaped. The changes in shape may be responsible for the heavier vaginal discharge women have after they have been pregnant. Your vagina also may be a little larger than it was prepregnancy, and if you are very body-aware you might notice that the labia are softer and fleshier.

Baby or not, all women in their 30s should make sure they have regular pap smear tests. The risk of developing the beginning stages of cervical cancer increases with age, especially if you smoke and your diet is poor. Up to half of all cervical abnormalities do return to normal without treatment, but some get worse quickly and need urgent treatment. Getting a pap smear result that indicates abnormal cell growth can be frightening, but if pap smear tests are taken regularly the disease will be detected in its infancy and can be safely and effectively treated.

Almost every woman will have a yeast infection at some time in her life and many of us are susceptible in our 30s. Yeast infections first make their presence felt by a burning, itching sensation and an increase in vaginal discharge, as well as pain with urination and during intercourse. Anything that disrupts the pH balance or bacterial balance of the vagina can result in infection. Repeated sexual intercourse over a short period of time; wearing restrictive, nonabsorbent, synthetic clothing close to the skin; chemical irritants, such as bubble bath; colored toilet paper, deodorants, leaving tampons in for more than eight hours, hot pools, and douches may also contribute to infection. Oral contraceptives and pregnancy can alter the acidity and sugar content of vaginal secretions. Other factors that can contribute to yeast infections include diabetes, the use of antibiotics, nutritional deficiencies, allergies, improper hygiene, and the consumption of refined carbohydrates. Some women are especially vulnerable to infection following their menstrual periods.

Decrease your intake of sugar if you have a yeast infection, to give the yeast less to feed on. Avoid sugar, fruit, refined carbohydrates, and sweets of any kind until the infection has healed. Also avoid alcohol, aged cheeses, fermented foods, mushrooms, yeast, and diary products, except for low-fat yogurt. Maintain the health of your immune system. Get proper rest, eat healthily, and get moderate exercise. Avoid stress and antibiotics. Keep the vaginal area clean and dry and wear loose-fitting cotton underwear. Most cases of vaginal infection can be treated by over-the-counter preparations. Some women find relief by douching with white vinegar or fresh garlic juice in a quart of warm water. This is the least expensive and least invasive way to treat yeast infections. The vinegar douche restores a clean, refreshed feeling since it clears out the irritating yeast. If there is no improvement in two weeks see a doctor.

Sexually Transmitted Diseases

If you are sexually active in your 30s, there is no guarantee that you will avoid exposure to sexually transmitted diseases. Your defenses are good health and a functional immune system as well as condoms, discrimination in your choice of partners, and practicing safe sex as best as you can until you can make a monogamous commitment.

It is important to detect sexually transmitted diseases in their early stages so that prompt treatment can begin, and, in the case of some diseases, damage to the body can be prevented. Here's a review of the early symptoms for some of the numerous diseases that are passed on either exclusively or primarily through sexual contact. Yeast infections, like candidiasis, can be passed on by sexual contact, but there are other causes (see the previous section).

- *AIDS (Acquired Immune Deficiency Syndrome)*—Headaches, night sweats, weight loss, swollen lymph glands, fever, swollen tongue and mouth, yeast infections, diarrhea, lung infections.
- *Genital herpes*—Itching, burning in the genital area, discomfort when urinating, a watery vaginal or urethal discharge, weeping, fluid filled eruptions in the vagina.
- *Genital warts*—Soft, cauliflower-like growths appearing either singly or in clusters in or around the vagina, anus, groin.
- *Gonorrhea*—Frequent, painful urination, cloudy vaginal discharge, vaginal itching, inflammation of the pelvic area, rectal discharge, abnormal uterine bleeding.

- *PID (Pelvic Inflammatory Disease)*—A pus-filled vaginal discharge with fever and lower abdominal pain.
- *Syphilis*—A sore on the genitalia, rash, patches of flaking tissue, fever, sore throat, sores in the mouth or anus.
- *Trichomoniasis*—Vaginal itching and pain with a foamy, greenish or yellow foul-smelling discharge.

If you think that you may have a sexually transmitted disease, seek medical advice immediately.

Your Thirtysomething Hair

The changes that occur in hair growth as you get older mystify scientists. For some reason growth of hair on the scalp and underarms decreases, but hair growth in other places like the ears, nostrils, and eyebrows often increases. In general, though, body hairs become less numerous. Changes in color and growth patterns also occur. Studies have shown that we shed about 100 hairs a day on average, but that hair density, diameter, and breaking strength decreases with age. Coarser hair percentage decreases and finer hair percentage increases.

Graying of the hair is probably the most conspicuous sign of getting older. "It can make a woman feel she has aged ten years in an instant" (Hutton, p. 48). Youth seems very far away and old age very near. Gray hair is by no means universal, and it does not occur at the same time in all people. Gray hair is caused by the loss of melanin-producing cells and the consequent loss of melanin. Melanin, produced by cells in the hair, is a pigment that gives color to the hair and skin. Graying, should it occur, usually begins at the temples, then extends to the top of the scalp.

Technically, gray hair does not exist. It is white hair mixing in with normal hair that gives it its characteristic appearance. Hair seems genetically programmed to turn white at a certain age. For some women this can be as early as 35, for others 50, for others 80. But it's a rare woman who doesn't have some white hairs by the age of 50.

There are many myths about gray hair, all of which are untrue. You won't go gray overnight if you have a tremendous shock. Two white hairs won't grow in the place of the one you plucked out. Gray hair is not thicker than your normal hair. Some experts believe that gray hair is an indicator of poor health, but so far there is no conclusive evidence to support this belief.

Many women in their 30s confronted with gray hairs said that they have problems managing it. That suddenly their hair was difficult to style. That hair seemed to lack its luster and glow. Shampoos that once made it shine don't work anymore. Visits to the hairdresser become more frequent.

Whether you have any gray hair or not there is no doubt that thirtysomething hair looks, acts, and feels different from the way it did when you were 20. There is much that you can do, however, to improve it, and this will be discussed in Part Three.

Thirtysomething Teeth

"I never thought I'd say this. I must be getting old. I actually floss every day now." (Victoria, age 35)

In your 30s, you may notice that teeth gradually discolor and gums recede with wear and tear. Gum disease can also flare up later in life, making your gums bleed and your breath smell bad. Gum disease attacks the tiny ligaments which surround the tooth roots and secure your teeth to the underlying jaw bone. Plaque bacteria attached to the neck of the tooth at the gum margin causes inflammation and bleeding and eventually allows the bacteria to penetrate down to the ligaments. If the problem is not caught in time the ligaments will become inflamed and the teeth will loosen.

Gum disease is caused by poor oral hygiene, poor health, and

124

poor diet. Vigorous brushing often makes the problem worse. Women in their 30s need to take special care of their teeth and observe proper dental hygiene to prevent their mouths from becoming badly damaged in later life (see Part Three).

Senses in the 30s

"Taken for granted until they threaten to desert us, all five senses dim slightly as we get older" (Hutton, p. 126).

For most women, the ability to hear higher sound frequencies begins to diminish in the 30s. The diminution in ability to hear high notes is accompanied by a decreased ability to hear louder sounds. Despite this, however, many of the women I talked to said that they couldn't tolerate loud noise any more. That they felt their hearing had gotten more sensitive.

"I go into a restaurant or a bar and if the music is too loud I just have to leave. It never used to worry me before. Kids who drive their cars with the radio blasting out really irritate me too. As I get older I can't tolerate loud noise anymore." (Carolyn, age 36)

Few things can be as isolating as the gradual loss of hearing. The fashion of having personal stereos constantly thumping and loud music playing has partly been blamed for hearing loss. It is difficult to hear high notes first and to distinguish what people are saying in a crowded room. Tinnitus is a high pitched noise that you carry around with you 24 hours a day. No one is really quite sure what causes it. It can appear by itself or as a symptom of another disorder, such as infection or noise-induced hearing loss.

Hopefully in your 30s hearing loss won't be a problem, but to prevent it from occurring, now is the time to start protecting your ears from damage by avoiding loud, sudden noises and walking around with earphones all the time.

Although not a sense organ, some women notice a change in their voices. They say that it isn't so easy to reach the high notes anymore, but that their voices sounded deeper, richer, more mature.

125

You may find in your 30s as your taste buds fully mature that you start liking foods you detested as a child. I always detested mustard but found it tolerable in my 30s. The ability to detect the four primary tastes (salt, sweet, sour, bitter) does decrease over time by a very small amount, but it is unlikely to do so in your 30s.

Your sense of smell, however, is more likely to decline in the 30s. Studies have shown that the loss of ability to detect odors begins to appear much earlier than other sensory losses. Diminished performance in odor detection has been found to begin in the early 20s. Those who use their sense of smell more than others, wine tasters for example, say that their sense of smell hadn't changed. It may just be a case of "use it or lose it" as far as smells are concerned.

It is changes in the lens of the eye that come closest to being a universal normal age change in humans. Your lenses become thicker and heavier with age, reducing the ability to focus on close-up objects. You may find as you edge toward your fortieth birthday that your arms aren't long enough anymore for you to focus on reading material. You need reading glasses.

To those who have never had to rely on glasses, this can come as a nasty shock. Those who have been shortsighted may enjoy a period when they can actually see better before needing bifocals. The eye, like the rest of you, is getting less supple as you age and less able to change focus quickly. When focusing distance becomes longer than the length of your arms, you have presbyopia. There seems to be nothing you can do about it, although vitamin A and other supplements may prove beneficial.

Bifocal glasses and contact lenses are available. It is possible to get reading glasses now without visible lines dividing the top and bottom of the lens which was always such an outward sign of age. Other vision problems are glaucoma and cataracts, but they tend to begin in the 40s. If you get yourself tested every six months in your mid-30s you should be able to control the development of any of these problems.

Some believe that eye exercises begun in the 20s and 30s can prevent presbyopia to some degree. Your doctor or optometrist may recommend someone who can teach you or you can learn about them from a book like *Better Sight Without Glasses* by Harry Benjamin, which was first published in 1929. Mr. Benjamin recommends the "Bates method," which is a series of focal distance changes called "swaying and palming." Stretching the neck and a "sensible naturopathic diet" are also recommended. For patients with presbyopia, Bates recommends 15 minutes of palming twice a day and then eye muscle exercises, followed by reading a newspaper as near as possible without straining. The eye muscle exercises include holding up the index finger of the right hand about 8 inches in front of the eyes, then looking from the finger to any large object 10 or more feet away.

Sleep

As you get older there will be changes in the amount of sleep you need. In your 20s, about the first 80 minutes of sleep is in the non-rapid eye movement (NREM) state. Rapid eye movement (REM) sleep then occurs, and the two states alternate about every 90 to 100 minutes. The older you get the more time you spend in the NREM sleep stage.

The amount of time spent in REM sleep seems to correlate with general well-being. This accounts for increased amounts of wakefulness when we try to fall asleep and the number of times we wake up when we have fallen asleep. Studies have also shown that as we get older we can be wakened more easily from sleep with bright lights or loud noises. You may find that you don't sleep so deeply anymore, and don't always wake feeling refreshed.

Recently it has been found that disturbances in breathing or respiration also increase. Snoring almost always indicates an abnormality somewhere in the breathing airway. Snoring affects your health because it means you are not sleeping well and not getting the oxygen you need to the brain. Overweight people with difficulty breathing often snore. There may even be sleep apnea, which wakes them up many times in the night. Snoring also means that not enough blood is getting to the brain. So snores should be checked out by a doctor.

Although getting enough quality sleep is important in our 30s for optimum health, getting too much sleep can cause problems too. It's important to find a balance that is right for you. "I used to love lying in bed until midday in my twenties, but now I'm in my thirties, if I stay in bed too long I get headaches," notes Sam, age 34. In our teens and 20s our bodies needed more sleep, but in our 30s our sleep needs decrease because there is not as much growth and activity going on at a cellular level. Too much sleep will make us feel out of condition.

Physiological Processes That Decline with Age

There is no denying the fact that in your 30s certain physiological processes will decline. Metabolic rate goes down. Maximum aerobic capacity decreases, and bone mass is also lost. All these many changes affect nutritional requirements, which also decrease in the 30s. In the Baltimore Longitudinal Study on Aging it was found that the optimum energy intake of 2,700 calories a day at age 30 declined to 2,100 a day at age 80. Calorific needs decrease especially when there is a decline in physical activity.

As body fat increases, protein or lean body mass decreases at about 6 pounds per decade from early adulthood. Most of the lean tissue loss represents lost muscle mass. Between the ages of 30 and 80 muscle strength decreases by about 30 percent. Grip strength is a good example. In women grip strength gradually declines with age.

However, we don't have to let that happen. Some physiological processes that naturally decline over the years can be modified with exercise and physical conditioning. We can improve cardiac efficiency, pulmonary function, and bone calcium levels; we can reduce body fat and increase our metabolic rate. The answer lies in physical and mental activity.

Lethargy and inactivity will accelerate the decline of physiological process. Lethargy is a lack of enthusiasm for anything, a lack of interest in life. Inactivity and lethargy often go hand in hand with depression and illness. If you do feel lethargic it might be worth looking at your diet and lifestyle. Are you getting enough exercise? Are you eating foods that can energize you? Are you sleeping enough? Are you enjoying your life? Nothing will age you faster than a life that is without enjoyment.

Activity, both physical and mental, will delay the aging process. It really is a case of "use it or lose it" in your 30s. Women who look youthful have energy and vitality in abundance. They are never lethargic.

So far we have covered almost every aspect of bodily health in the 30s, but one vital piece of the puzzle needs to be discussed in more detail. What is happening to your hormones?

Chapter 6
Hormones

Our hormones begin fluctuating when we reach 30. By the time we are in our late 30s they will have already begun to drop in preparation for menopause. The processes of perimenopause and menopause in the next chapter. For now we'll take a look at how hormones function and discuss the roles hormones play in menstruation, childbearing, and emotional health.

Hormones

The word hormone is derived from the Greek word "hormonal," which means "I arouse to activity." A hormone is a biochemical messenger that is basically a call to action. It can work with incredible speed, complexity, and specificity to communicate information. "I think of hormones as chemical communicators or connectors," writes Dr. Elizabeth Lee Vliet in *Screaming to be Heard*, "that carry messengers to and from all organs of the body and serve to connect one organ's function with another organ's function to keep the body balanced and functioning normally" (1995, p. 35).

A correct balance of hormones is crucial for good health and normal adult development. Hormones regulate the body's functions and are necessary for life. The way you look, grow, feel, act, learn, the way your body digests food, grows hair, maintains its temperature, eliminates waste, and develops is all dependent on hormones. Even the functions of some hormones themselves are regulated by other hormones.

So when the levels of certain hormones are too high or too low, or when the body reacts to hormones in an unusual way, we won't feel so good. According to some experts we are also likely to age faster. "If anything goes wrong with that complex hormonal communication system," writes Barry Sears in *The Anti-Aging Zone,* "you begin to age far faster than you should" (p. 257). According to Sears the real foundation of aging is hormonal miscommunication. It is believed that increased hormonal miscommunication occurs with increasing age. The way, then, to try to defy age is to decrease hormonal miscommunication. Sears and many others believe this can be done through diet and stress reduction. Other experts believe that hormonal therapy is the answer.

Should hormonal imbalance occur in your 30s, more often than not it tends to be caused by the following different but interconnected hormone systems:

- Blood sugar hormones such as insulin and glucagon, which regulate blood sugar.
- Adrenal hormones, which include stress and sex hormones.
- Ovarian hormones such as estrogen and progesterone, the sex hormones.
- Thyroid hormones, which enhance the action of insulin and adrenal stress hormone.

You need only to look at these hormone groups to see that there has to be a relationship between nutrition, stress, and sex hormones. Many of us in our 30s would feel a lot healthier if we ate a balanced diet, reduced stress, and exercised regularly. These self-help measures have been shown to restore the body to a state of hormonal balance.

Sex Hormones—Estrogen, Progesterone, and Androgen

The sex hormones estrogen, progesterone, and testosterone, the most powerful form of androgen, act on our brain to regulate the menstrual cycle. If these hormones are in balance there should be no problem with the menstrual cycle. If they are not in balance, menstrual cycle irregularity will occur and you could experience symptoms similar to those of perimenopause and menopause.

The effects of estrogen deficiency in women have been well documented because they occur at menopause. Irregular or absent periods, reduction in breast size, poor vision, tooth and hair loss, vaginal dryness, frequent urination, risk of colon cancer, muddled thinking, depression, hot flashes, osteoporosis, and heart disease are all related to lowered estrogen levels. If estrogen levels are too low the walls of the vagina get too thin and there may also be a lack of lubrication. This could make intercourse painful. The hormone also has a wider effect on the whole body. Secretions and deposits of body fat are all dependent on estrogen. It influences blood proteins, fats, and the production of blood vessels and bones.

Estrogen levels that are too high in relation to progesterone levels can also cause problems. Estrogen dominance can accelerate the aging process. Symptoms include depression, weight gain, fatigue, headaches, PMS, loss of libido, bloating, mood swings, and breast tenderness.

When progesterone levels are too low periods are heavy and prolonged. Lack of progesterone increases the risk of cancer in the long term, because the endometrial cells do not progress to their proper mature form. Progesterone also has effects elsewhere on the body to prepare it for pregnancy. These are familiar to all women because they are experienced in the second half of the menstrual cycle. Fluid retention occurs in order to increase blood volume. Weight gain provides a store of nutrition for the fetus, and there is stimulation of the breast, producing an increase in size and often a degree of tenderness. Because progesterone acts on the brain, changes in mood are often experienced in the later part of the cycle. Too little progesterone and your mood will drop in the PMS despair so familiar to many.

Estrogen and progesterone are commonly thought of as the "female hormones." But it should be pointed out that estrogen is present in men and is made in the testicle, and androgens, the so-called male hormones of which testosterone is the most powerful, play an essential role in female development. Androgens belong in a woman's body as much as in a man's. They are of tremendous benefit to women. They affect every tissue and play a crucial role in making the body function normally and are particularly important to the health of bones and muscles and the reproductive cycle.

In order to feel well it is important to maintain the small but essential amount of androgen hormone that is right for you. If levels fall too low you may notice that your muscles lose tone, that your hair loses shine, your skin loses its glow. If on the other hand levels rise too high you could develop menstrual irregularity, acne, increased facial hair, scalp hair loss, and be at increased risk of infertility, heart disease, and diabetes. One in ten women is affected by androgen disorders and they often are not diagnosed properly because the symptoms may appear unrelated.

Androgen disorders, when the adrenal and ovarian glands over-produce androgen hormones, tend to affect women in their 30s. This is why medical textbooks usually state that women in their 30s are most prone to the disorder. This is not entirely accurate. You can have an androgen disorder at any age. Most likely to be noticed in the 30s, the disorder has been there since puberty, but ignored because symptoms were mild. The pill tends to suppress androgen-like symptoms and is the most common form of treatment offered by doctors.

Now let's look at the many facets of life that are affected by our fluctuating hormones—from menstrual rhythms to sexuality and childbearing.

Irregular Periods

Many women in their 30s notice that as they get older their periods get shorter. Irregular and unusual periods are not uncommon. To understand why irregular and lighter periods are so common in the 30s we first need to understand what happens during a normal menstrual cycle.

The menstrual cycle occurs every 28 or 29 days on average, with day one being the first day of your period. The first part of the menstrual cycle up to ovulation is called the follicular phase, when estrogen is dominant. The endometrial lining in the uterus builds up now, ready to receive and nourish an egg should fertilization occur. In the ovary one or two eggs are being prepared for ovulation. Every time a woman ovulates hundreds of eggs are used up but only one or two will fully mature. The rest will die. As we get older we use up eggs more rapidly and in her 30s the average woman uses around 50,000 eggs.

A mid-cycle surge in hormones, including testosterone, triggers the release of an egg. It will burst out of the ovary and move into the waiting fallopian tube. At the place on the ovary where the egg was released, the corpus luteum is formed, which produces progesterone during the second half of the cycle, called the luteal phase. Progesterone continues to prepare the womb for pregnancy or menstruation should conception not occur. Estrogen is produced throughout the whole cycle, but it is more dominant in the first half. Progesterone is low or absent in the first half of the cycle but dominant in the second.

In our 20s the hormones that regulate the menstrual cycle tend to be in balance. For example, estrogen levels tend to be similar throughout our cycles, but as we get older levels begin to fluctuate, making PMS, heavy periods, light periods, and long delays between periods more likely. Each month as eggs are used up hormone levels start to change. The result is that our periods get more and more unpredictable. If there is too much estrogen, for instance, periods can be too heavy. If there is too little periods will be light. If androgen levels are too high ovulation will be suppressed and periods absent.

Many of us assume that menstrual problems are natural. That problems, pain, and discomfort are to be endured. But the truth is that this is not so. The menstrual cycle is very sensitive and can easily be upset by stress, drugs, excessive dieting, overexercise, poor diet, and illness. In most cases the problem can be remedied with stress reduction, a sensible diet, and exercise and weight management, but in more severe cases hormonal therapy will be needed.

PMS

"Women who are going through PMS can lead pretty miserable lives for part of every month," writes Gillian Ford in *Listening to Your Hormones* (1997, p. 117). To say you have premenstrual syndrome, or PMS, is to announce to the world that you feel moody, anxious, irritable, ugly, and fat. In short, you don't feel youthful and energetic and you don't feel up to doing much. You feel old.

PMS tends to strike more women in their 30s than in their teens and 20s. Experts believe that there are a number of reasons why this is so. Women in their 30s are more prone to hormonal swings caused by pregnancy, breastfeeding, miscarriage, and going on and off the pill. PMS could be caused by the fact that hormonal imbalance has driven progesterone levels too low and, as progesterone is believed to have a soothing effect, the result is tension, irritability, and anxiety. Other researchers believe that women in their 30s have higher stress levels than before and that stress plays a large part in the development of the disorder.

PMS, despite the fact that up to 90 percent of women in their reproductive years experience it in some form, is still considered to be a controversial syndrome. Experts have differing opinions about what causes it. Explanations range from hormonal imbalance like low progesterone levels and the body's inability to handle an imbalance of estrogen and progesterone, to nutritional deficiencies like vitamin B_6 and magnesium deficiency, to psychological factors such as stress. Experts are undecided about whether or not PMS is a medical condition or not.

Whatever medical experts think, a woman with PMS knows that

she is feeling out of sorts and that the condition is robbing her of her youthful vitality. What she wants to know is what she can do about it to keep symptoms minimal. Following are a few suggestions, but if symptoms are severe, make sure you go and see a doctor for advice.

First of all, don't just put up with the problem if it is destroying the quality of your life. PMS is not an inevitable part of being a woman and something that has to be endured. You can do something about it.

Make sure that you have PMS and that your problem is caused by hormones rather than other factors in your life. To be diagnosed with PMS, symptoms need to occur in two out of three menstrual cycles. Keeping track of exactly when in your cycle you feel premenstrual will help you know if you really have PMS and help you prepare for it when it comes. Warn family and friends that your health may be poor around that time.

Take note of exactly what your symptoms are so that you can learn more about them and how to deal with them. Make sure that you eat a healthy diet. Cut down on too much salt, fat, sugar, alcohol, nicotine, and caffeine, all of which can make PMS worse. Estrogen and progesterone derive from cholesterol, so the right fat intake is important for hormone balance. Increase the consumption of essential fatty acids to metabolize hormones. Evening primrose oil, borage oil, and flaxseed oil are good sources. Boosting your calcium intake may also prove to be beneficial, as studies have shown that increased calcium intake can ease symptoms of PMS. All that may be required is an extra cup of skim milk or yogurt. Try to keep your blood sugar levels stable by eating frequent small meals. You might consider taking vitamin supplements of B complex, especially B_6 and B_{12}, and vitamin E. Some believe that magnesium deficiency may be associated with PMS. Some women have found relief with dong quai, an aromatic herb grown in China, Korea, and Japan. Black cohosh and chasteberry also have calming effects.

Make sure you exercise. Women who exercise regularly find that symptoms of PMS are alleviated. Include relaxation in your daily routine. You could well find that simply relaxing more eases symptoms. And finally, you might benefit from using natural progesterone cream, like Pro-Gest, which is available without prescription. It can be especially helpful in the second half, the luteal phase, of your cycle. You may need to use it for two or three monthly cycles before you notice a difference in your symptoms.

Endometriosis

Endometriosis affects millions of women in America in their 30s. It is debilitating and painful and will make you feel older than you are. What causes it is endometrial tissue, which is similar to tissue from the lining of the uterus, that grows outside the uterine cavity. It can cause cramping, pain, and discomfort before and during a period, and if left untreated increases the risk of infertility. Depending on where the tissue has grown it can cause pain when you go to the restroom or when you are having sex.

Some women have mild symptoms, but others have chronic pain that can slowly wear them down. You also won't know if your fertility is affected until you try to get pregnant. As endometriosis can cause infertility, this can be a source of great distress.

Some experts believe that endometriosis is stress related. Stress levels are often very high for women in their 30s, especially those who are juggling work and family responsibilities. But too much can be made of the stress connection. Certainly it may contribute to the development of the disorder, but it also encourages self-blame, which can make the condition worse. It appears that there could be a genetic predisposition to the disorder.

The condition can be diagnosed through a surgical procedure called a laparoscopy and treated with surgery or drugs. Unfortunately, these drugs can have unpleasant side effects. A drastic remedy is a hysterectomy. Endometriosis is a very common reason for women in their 30s to have a hysterectomy.

Once it has set in, endometriosis seems to be unpreventable, but there are things you can do to stop the discomfort wearing you down. Learning about your condition and accepting that it is going to be a part of your life may help you find what works best with you. Exercising, eating healthily, cutting down on too much fat and sugar—especially chocolate—may help. Applying heat to areas of pain can alleviate some of the discomfort. You can try over-the-counter medications for relief, or if these don't help, ask your doctor. Going on the pill can also relieve symptoms. Reducing your stress levels is important. If sex is painful, focus more on intimacy and hugging. And finally, seek support. Find a self-help group where you can talk to other sufferers.

Polycystic Ovaries

Women with higher than normal levels of androgen hormone tend to have menstrual cycles that are anovulatory. This means that they do not ovulate. No egg is released from the ovary because the androgen levels suppress ovulation. If your periods are very irregular, it is highly likely that you are not ovulating.

How anovulation affects every woman will vary. Some will stop menstruating altogether, others will still have infrequent bleeding, others will have heavy periods that are longer than usual. All will be temporarily infertile. Women who have anovulatory cycles usually go on to develop a disorder known as polycystic ovary syndrome or PCOS.

When excessive androgens inhibit follicular development and cysts develop in the ovaries to produce even more androgen, this condition is called polycystic ovary syndrome or PCOS. PCOS is the most common cause of menstrual irregularity. PCOS is an extremely complicated disorder in which excess androgen from the adrenals and ovaries causes the brain to send confusing signals to the ovaries. Follicles start to mature but fail to ripen properly. The eggs are not released at the appropriate time, but they stay in the ovary and continue to make hormones so that even more androgen is circulating in the body. Over time more and more trapped follicles build up in the ovaries so that they become filled with hard fibrotic growths or cysts. Without ovulation normal menstrual function cannot occur. The most sensitive test for PCOS is a transvaginal ultrasound. The characteristic appearance of PCOS is a ring of small to medium follicles around the circumference of an enlarged ovary.

Usually this condition begins just before puberty, but it takes time to develop and the polycystic appearance of the ovaries may not be detected until the 20s or 30s when symptoms become more severe. Prior to that symptoms probably manifest in a mild way but are ignored and dismissed because they seem so mild—the odd missed period or bout of acne past puberty. Weight gain, male hair growth, acne, irregular periods, infertility, and increased risk of cancer of the lining of the uterus are also associated with PCOS.

Symptoms of PCOS range from the mild to the severe. The condition is still poorly understood, but some experts believe that a genetic predisposition to androgen excess may be the case. Daughters of patients with PCOS seem at higher risk of getting the disease. Other doctors believe that there is a strong connection between insulin resistance and the development of PCOS.

Unfortunately PCOS seems to be a condition that doesn't fade with time. More often than not it gets worse. Eating sensibly, managing your weight, exercising regularly, and reducing the amount of stress in your life will alleviate symptoms, even if it will not cure them. Doctors will recommend hormonal therapy.

Hypothalamic Amenorrhea— Severe Estrogen Deficiency

Some cases of absent periods are caused by a condition known as hypothalamic amenorrhea. It differs from anovulation due to androgen excess because in the latter case the cycle starts normally and estrogen is produced but somehow falters at ovulation. With hypothalamic amenorrhea the cycle never starts at all, and severe estrogen deficiency is likely.

The condition is often caused by high levels of stress, which cause the hypothalamus to malfunction. The hypothalamus is thought to be the master control center for the reproductive cycle, determining when the correct hormonal signals should be sent via the pituitary gland to the ovaries. The stress can be any kind. Moving to a new house, changing jobs, grieving for a loved one, a poor diet, too much exercise, gaining or losing too much weight can all put the body in a state of crisis and cause skipped periods. Usually, once stress is reduced through relaxation, diet, exercise, and weight gain or loss, normal reproductive functions return.

In some cases, though, periods don't return. This is often the case when stress has continued for many years without relief, when there are long-term eating disorders or when there is an exhaustive exercise program. All these triggers can seriously upset the hormonal balance of the body. If the periods don't return, however, hormonal therapy is advised. Premature menopause, osteoporosis, and infertility are associated with severe estrogen deficiency. If your periods have been absent for more than three months and you know you are not pregnant, make sure you go and see a doctor.

Sexuality

There is little doubt that our hormones affect how we feel about ourselves sexually. If our hormones are not in balance we won't feel good, and if health is poor sex often suffers. Too little estrogen, for example, can cause vaginal dryness. An excess of androgen hormone can cause problems with skin and hair, which can be inhibiting.

If we lead a healthy lifestyle and pay attention to our stress levels, hormones in the 30s should not be causing us too much discomfort, unless severe symptoms of perimenopause or menopause have already set in. Most women report that sex in the 30s gets better and better. Even if there are physiological changes with age—skin flushes less luridly, breasts don't get quite so engorged, blood flow to the vagina diminishes slightly—this in no way impairs enjoyment. Sensations may be less intense, but instead they are more prolonged, allowing for more leisurely enjoyment. And many women report that sensations are more intense because they enjoy sex more. We know our bodies better and our levels of confidence, both in our bodies and in our abilities to survive in the world, are higher than they were in our 20s.

Despite this, other changes may lead us to feel anxious about our sexuality, even if we are not affected by aging. Many of us still feel attractive but wonder if we are losing something.

"I don't know what I've lost. Just being noticed I think. I don't want unwelcome sexual attention anymore, but I also don't want to be easily forgotten. I get ignored more now I'm in my thirties." (Tracy, age 34)

In our 30s our enjoyment of sex may intensify, but leaving the high visibility of youth behind can be like losing a kind of power. We may realize for the first time how powerful our sexual attractiveness was in our teens and 20s—now just as we see it ebbing away from us. We know we shouldn't be obsessed about physical changes. That as strong women we don't need to judge ourselves by shallow cultural standards. That the idea that men get better with age while women just get old is just an idea foisted on us by our culture. Yet a part of us may still pine for the high visibility of youth. If this is the case, rethinking our definition of attractiveness, realizing that younger women tend to get more attention not because they look more attractive but because they look more vulnerable, and cultivating a positive body image are ways to increase our sexual confidence and pleasure.

Contraception

Studies show that up to the age of 35 women take contraception very seriously. After that the reverse happens. We stop believing we can have babies. Our fertility does fall off after 35, but our ovaries are in no way ready to be retired. Every woman is highly individual, but most of us will continue to ovulate until periods stop, which is from the late 40s up to the early 50s.

A relaxed attitude to contraception is common in the mid-to-late 30s. Some of us switch to the rhythm method, which is highly unreliable because this is the decade when periods start getting more and more irregular. Contrary to popular belief, unwanted pregnancies happen more the older we get. More abortions are carried out for women in their 30s than in any other decade. On the positive side, though, those of us who do use contraception in our 30s have lower failure rates because we are more conscientious about taking or using them correctly.

One of the most effective forms of contraception is the pill, but many women in their mid-30s stop taking it. Pill usage declines dramatically in the over-30 age group. There is concern about the possible side effects that have been rumored to be associated with the pill—weight gain, infertility, depression, and increased risk of heart attack.

The pill will always be controversial. It causes women to walk about in an altered biochemical state. Even Sir Charles Dobbs, the scientist who synthesized orally effective estrogen in 1938, lived to deplore the application of his discovery. "When a clock is working," he said gloomily, "you don't tinker with it." For those interested in the great pill debate, Barbara Seaman's *The Doctor's Case Against the Pill* (1995) is sobering. On the other hand, the pill has many supporters. Some argue that the pill, by suppressing regular ovulation, makes modern women's bodies mimic women's bodies in earlier centuries when women were pregnant or breast-feeding much of the time and therefore not ovulating. The pill is also thought to protect against tumors and cysts and to correct certain hormonal disorders, like androgen excess.

The pill is not thought to be dangerous if taken a long time. According to a ruling by the Food and Drug Administration in 1989 a healthy, nonsmoking woman can take it right up to menopause. The pill has revolutionized women's lives and taken away the fear of unwanted pregnancy. The evidence to take it is persuasive, but many of us in our 30s are still undecided. Only one in a hundred women takes it.

Make sure you take one of the newer, safer, lower-dose options if you do decide to go on or continue taking the pill. One of these is the combined pill which contains both estrogen and progestin. The hormone dose is low and daily estrogen levels included in the pill have been cut back dramatically. There are fewer side effects and health risks. Since the 1980s, a new kind of progestin used for the pill has changed the picture. Although not completely devoid of side effects, it is a great improvement.

With new lower-dose estrogen pills, fears that the pill would cause breast and cervical cancer have been laid to rest. Studies have shown that the risk of breast cancer for pill takers after the age of 25 is minimal. The pill also seems to have a protective effect against ovarian cancer and cancer of the endometrium. Risk of heart attack only increases if you smoke. Smoking when you are on the pill is dangerous at any age. Smoking prevents the extra estrogen from having a beneficial action on substances that help dissolve blood clots.

The pill has other benefits in the 30s. It can be a great help if you suffer from irregular periods, premenstrual syndrome, or androgen disorder. Because it regularizes the menstrual cycle it can also be an effective form of hormonal therapy for various hormonal imbalances, as well as symptoms of perimenopause.

The pill will probably always be a controversial drug. If you are undecided, take time to read up on and research the pill. Talk to your doctor about your concerns. Most doctors will assure you that the pill is probably one of the most researched medications in history. If you don't smoke and don't have cardiovascular risk factors, which include a parent or sibling having a stroke under the age of 45, marked obesity, diabetes, high blood pressure, or abnormal levels of blood fats, the pill is probably a safe form of contraception in your 30s. Bear in mind, though, that there are hundreds of hormones involved in the menstrual cycle and the pill only mimics two. The safety of the pill depends on which experts you listen to and each woman's individual tolerance of it.

Once you are in your 30s you may find that your doctor wants you to consider progestin-only methods of hormonal contraception, as the absence of estrogen removes the slight risk to circulation. The progestin pill is taken continuously at the same time each day and works by changing the cervical mucus, making it more impenetrable to sperm. It may even stop ovulation. Other doctors, however, are more reluctant to deprive you of bone-preserving and heart-protecting estrogen.

A form of contraception that became increasingly popular for women in their 30s was the injectable contraception also known as Depo Provera or DMPA. Progestin-only implants can provide contraception for up to five years. Made up of six flexible rods, they are inserted into the upper arm under local anesthetic where they continue to be visible. A slow-release progestin seeps into the blood stream. Progestin can also be injected every few months or inserted into the vagina by a ring. The injections or implants were once considered to be totally safe and not to affect fertility, but since the 1970s injectable contraception has received much criticism. Many experts believe that there are health risks, such as osteoporosis, breast cancer, and infertility, and are withdrawing them from use. Norplant is no longer available. There are reports coming from women who wanted their implants out but they are proving harder to remove than previously thought.

The intra-uterine device (IUD) is making a cautious comeback among women in their 30s. It is extremely popular in Europe for women over 30. The new generation of IUDs can be painful when fitted, but the majority need changing only every five years or so. There are few side effects (abnormal bleeding and painful, heavy periods) and today the risk of infection is minimal.

A surprising number of women in their 30s are abandoning the pill and other forms of hormonal contraception in their 30s and opting for natural family planning or barrier methods. Natural family planning requires time, patience, a lot of body awareness, and often a trained instructor if it is to be successful. Remember, though, that in our 30s our periods do tend to become more and more irregular, making it difficult to track ovulation and the potentially fertile period.

Using condoms not only provides the best protection against the risk of sexually transmitted disease and fatal illness but it also is an effective form of contraception which doesn't alter the chemical balance of your body. When used correctly condoms are comparable in effectiveness to the pill and because they don't alter the body's biochemical state this makes them automatically safer. Most women in their 30s agreed that condoms wouldn't have worked so well in the 20s. To carry them off you need a sense of humor, a certain degree of confidence, and hopefully a good relationship—all of which are more likely in your 30s. Some women feel that using condoms takes way the spontaneity of love making, but putting on condoms can become part of erotic foreplay. Women in their 30s who used the diaphragm or Dutch cap also found that if used correctly it offers protection not only against pregnancy but also against sexually transmitted disease and cervical cancer.

After the age of 30, sterilization becomes a more popular option. By the early 40s, one-half of all couples has been sterilized, and it's usually the woman despite the fact that vasectomy is simpler and more easily reversed. Sterilization for women is a 20-minute operation where a small incision is made and the fallopian tubes are either tied or closed off so that eggs cannot travel down the tube and are reabsorbed by the body.

Sterilization was once thought to lead to hormonal imbalances characterized by difficult or irregular periods, loss of libido, vaginal dryness, and so on but there is no real evidence to suggest that this is the case. It is a drastic step to take in your 30s and I recommend it be seen as the final option before others have been explored. It is only suitable for those who are determined not to have more children or who don't want to have children at all because it is almost

100 percent irreversible. The 30s are the decade of transition and it is often hard to tell how we will feel about fertility, children, and family 5 years down the road. It was sad to talk to Linda, who opted for sterilization when she was 32. She's 36 now and two years ago passionately longed to have children. She tried to get her operation reversed but her fertility was not restored. However, there are also many women who remain perfectly happy with the decision.

Fertility

More and more women in their 30s are having babies. The trend is no longer to squeeze childbearing into the years of your reproductive prime, but to have babies later. In 1990, four times as many first babies were born to American women over the age of 30 as were born in 1970, and the number of first-time mothers in their 40s has doubled.

There are some of us in our early 30s who are panicky about pregnancy, but many more of us don't feel the urgency to reproduce. Sue, 35, says, "Every year I say to myself I should have babies now but every year I decide to wait another year. It's just not the right time."

Establishing a career, finding a sense of self, and embarking on motherhood with good health, good financial backing, and, in many cases, a stable relationship is a pattern that is becoming more and more common. With developments in modern health care many of us can afford to take our time. Even the medical profession is on our side. It says that having a baby in your 30s could actually be an advantage on the grounds that women in their 30s are probably in better shape than they were in their 20s, more likely to have established medical care, and more likely to cope with the demands and changes pregnancy brings.

Having a baby in your 30s tends to be more exhausting than if you were younger. The older you get the longer it takes to get in shape physically, and there is more likelihood of a weakened pelvic floor and all its attendant problems. Having lived an independent, organized life, it can be difficult to adjust to the chaos and dependency a baby brings. "I really liked my life. I had a routine. Baby has changed all that. I miss having times of quiet reflection. I miss being alone," says Tracy, who is 33 and the mother of Thomas, age 2.

Motherhood is exhausting whatever your age. Rearing a child is hard work, but the moms I spoke to in their 30s all tended to be quite relaxed. They enjoyed their babies, and more often than not were financially stable and in supportive relationships. They also had a clearer idea of what they want for their kids and how to bring them up.

On the other hand, the risks attached to pregnancy increase the longer you postpone it. You can face higher risks of miscarriage, infertility, and complications in genetic conditions. The array of prenatal tests and screenings recommended for older moms can be nerve wracking. Doctors tend to be perhaps overly cautious of the older pregnant woman, and C sections are often scheduled routinely.

Complications that are more likely as you get older include pregnancy-induced hypertension, which rises from 10 percent in the early 20s to 20 percent in the late 30s. Older women also have more chance of developing diabetes or a pronounced glucose intolerance, which carries a greater likelihood of complications. Heart disease and obesity, which can also complicate matters, are more common with age. Prenatal checks are the best way a pregnant woman can protect herself.

The possibility of genetic abnormalities was the greatest fear among the thirtysomething moms I talked to. Chromosomes don't divide as perfectly and the biggest problem is the missing 21st chromosome, an anomaly that results in Down's syndrome. The association of this condition with advancing maternal age is striking. According to several large studies, the incidence raises from about 1 in 1,350 in your 20s to 1 in 385 at 35 and 1 in 40 at 40.

Other studies are more hopeful and show that other birth defects like spina bifida have no relation to the mom's age. This may be reassuring to women in their 30s considering childbearing. The chances of a baby being born with a genetic abnormality have been greatly decreased by genetic diagnosis, which can identify certain conditions like cystic fibrosis or Down's syndrome. It is important that moms avail themselves of all the appropriate tests so that decisions can be made. It is also important that decisions are made as to the probable outcome before the tests are conducted. Amniocentesis is the procedure highly recommended for women over 35 but there is a slight risk of provoking miscarriage. Thankfully, detailed ultrasounds and biochemical blood tests for Down's syndrome are eliminating the need for amniocentesis in older moms.

The later you leave it to have a baby, the more you will be considered high risk by the medical profession. Should problems arise, talk with your doctor and consider all the options. And if no problems arise, which is far more likely, try not to let all the tests take away the enjoyment and excitement of your pregnancy.

Infertility

The biggest obstacle to motherhood for many of us in our 30s may be getting pregnant in the first place. This can be frustrating if in your 20s you got pregnant easily or had an abortion. Our fertility does start to decline on our thirtieth birthday, and strikingly so after the age of 35. In addition, the older you are the more likely you are to have suffered conditions like diabetes, stress, obesity, sexually transmitted disease, and stress, all of which can affect your fertility. A Dutch study showed that after the age of 31 fertility drops by 112 percent a year and a 35-year-old is twice as likely to have her pregnancy end in miscarriage as a 25-year-old.

What these kinds of studies may reveal though, is that it just takes longer for older women to conceive. Other studies show that with perseverance older women do conceive. A two-year delay before pregnancy can be hard for many of us who are all too aware of the biological clock. The stress caused by the fear of infertility often makes the situation worse, as infertility is known to be stress induced.

Christiane Northrup in *Women's Bodies, Women's Wisdom* (1997) shows that infertility may be caused by irregular ovulation, problems with the fallopian tubes, or endometriosis. Also, immunological problems may contribute as a woman makes antibodies that are resistant to her partner's sperm. Yet the factor that unites all categories is stress. "The question of whether stress causes infertility or infertility creates stress has been hotly debated with no scientific resolution," writes Joan Borysenko in *The Woman's Book of Life* (p. 108). But overwhelming evidence does seem to suggest that women who are having problems conceiving are usually highly stressed and that stress reduction should be an important part of treatment.

Older women take longer to conceive because they have more cycles when no eggs are produced. Eggs are released erratically, sometimes one, sometimes two (nonidentical twin births increase with age), and sometimes none at all. If attempts at fertility are disappointing, try using a home ovulation kit to predict exactly when you are at your most fertile. Managing your weight, eating sensibly, reducing stress, and exercising regularly will help too. If after six months to a year you are still having a problem, see an infertility specialist rather than your gynecologist, who does not specialize in infertility. Don't automatically think you are a candidate for IVF or donor eggs. Most infertility problems are resolved with simple fertility tests or lifestyle changes like weight management through diet and exercise. Ovulation drugs like clomid and pergonal have an extremely high success rate. Make sure you get your partner checked out too. You may not be the problem.

Statistics are giving hope to older moms, but the message still is that you shouldn't wait too long if you want children in your 30s and should consider conception as soon as your situation allows. As every year passes your fertility declines and a 3-year gap in your 30s while you decide can make a huge difference. After you hit 40, even if you have had children, fertility cannot be relied upon. The risk of miscarriage doubles in your early 40s, not because of the age of the uterus, but because of the age of your eggs.

In the future doctors hope to delay the aging process of the ovaries by slowing down the rate at which eggs are lost, so that our reproductive years can be extended by 10 or 20 years. Others talk of removing the womb and reimplanting it later so that women can suspend fertility. It is already possible to remove and freeze eggs to be used at a later date. In several years' time we may all be offered the option of freezing ovarian tissue. The merits of such drastic measures are dubious. It is wrong to think that a woman's worth is defined by whether she has children or not. Attempts to suspend the biological clock show just how much fear there is in our culture of leaving youth behind, of letting go of one phase in life and beginning another.

Hysterectomies

Hysterectomies are performed at a high rate in the United States and Canada. "Despite some better alternatives, hysterectomy is still one of the most common operations in the Western World" (Hutton, p. 184). Many of the operations to remove the uterus, ovaries, and fallopian tubes are attempts to remedy problems caused by hormonal imbalance.

The uterus, ovaries, and fallopian tubes were for centuries hidden from view, but even though modern medicine has taken away some of the mystery, many of us are still apprehensive and uneducated about our own reproductive system. Interestingly, the word *hysteria* comes from the Greek for "womb." At one time it was thought that the womb could wander around the body and it was responsible for madness and paranoia. Even today we blame mood swings, unpredictability, and depression on our reproductive system.

According to Christiane Northrup we rely too heavily on the advice of doctors and experts about our reproductive system and neglect our own intuition. Hysterectomy is understandable for cancer treatment, but all too often the operation is carried out for minor reasons simply because doctors believe that if a woman doesn't want babies anymore the womb may as well come out. The womb is considered to be useless except for childbearing. The problem with this drastic approach is that it leaves our bodies in a permanent state of hormonal imbalance without the ovaries, and also removes an organ that is not designed to disappear after menopause. We still don't know the functions of the womb after menopause, but it is possible that it carries with it certain health benefits.

Certainly the operation to have the uterus surgically removed is sometimes essential. If cancer is diagnosed there really is very little choice. The problem is that too often wombs are removed for far less serious conditions which could be treated by other less drastic methods. Hysterectomy for conditions like heavy bleeding, endometriosis, or fibroid tumors is getting harder to defend especially with less radical options now becoming available like endometrial ablation and laparoscopic (keyhole) surgery. These operations solve the problem while leaving the ovaries intact and are far less invasive than a hysterectomy.

"When it comes to aging, nothing can bring it on more abruptly than a hysterectomy in which the ovaries are removed" (*Prevention* editors, p. 158). There will be symptoms of menopause and an end to fertility. If you are in your 30s and considering a hysterectomy make sure you get a second, a third, and maybe even a fourth opinion. Make sure you explore all the options available to you.

Pregnancy and the Baby Blues

For many women the experience of pregnancy is a beautiful and fulfilling one. Sure there are discomforts, but these are to be expected. For other women, however, pregnancy may be an ordeal. Weight gain may cause anxiety. After years of dieting suddenly seeing your body swell can be scary. Morning sickness can be horrendous. Depression and mood swings can occur.

It makes sense that morning sickness and depression and anxiety are all related to the massive hormonal shifts taking place as your body prepares for new life. Unfortunately, though, as with many other female problems, doctors may not give you much sympathy and to make matters worse, everyone expects you to be pregnant and loving it. Making sure you get lots of rest, taking good care of yourself, eating sensibly, exercising regularly, and reducing stress are the best ways to fight prenatal blues.

Most new moms also experience some kind of mood instability in the first few weeks postpartum—one minute elated, the next weepy. You get impatient. You get irritable. You feel fat and out of shape. You don't seem to be able to control your moods. Giving birth and crossing over to motherhood is a challenging and emotional time. The first few weeks, months, and even years are a period of readjustment for you and your family. It's a myth that baby blues last only a few days after delivery. It can start during pregnancy as your body and your life start to transform. It can linger on for months postpartum. If you were used to routine, if you were used to freedom, if you were used to time alone, your whole world changes. Your baby will leave no part of your life untouched.

There is an explanation for the emotional twilight zone that occurs postpartum. Having a baby is emotionally exhausting. It is easy to feel overwhelmed. At no other time in your life will you lose weight so rapidly. At no other time in your life will your hormone levels drop so rapidly. It took your body nine months to prepare for your baby, and in about six weeks your body races to undo all that. Small wonder you are exhausted.

Feeling down after childbirth is a common experience for many women. It is important to give yourself and your hormones a chance to settle down. Don't expect your life to have routine and order for quite a while. Be patient with yourself. Help yourself by making sure you eat well and that you ease back into a gentle exercise routine. It is also important to talk to others about how you feel.

In contrast to the baby blues, which strikes within days after birth, postpartum depression (PPD) usually strikes a little later. It usually happens about two weeks after delivery and can last for months on end. There could be insomnia, aversion to the baby, fear of harming the baby, and loss of interest in life. PPD is a serious mood disorder which strikes about ten percent of new moms. It is due to a chemical imbalance in the brain which is aggravated by a drop in pregnancy hormones postpartum and the stress of motherhood. Postpartum depression is dangerous and if you feel that you have something far more serious than the baby blues, make sure you seek medical advice immediately.

Chronic Fatigue

In normal circumstances, the main hormonal systems that govern stress and sex hormones all strengthen immunity. So when there is hormonal imbalance the immune system is affected. Susceptibility to illness and fatigue are likely.

More and more women in their 30s are suffering from chronic fatigue syndrome (CFS). The Centers for Disease Control defines CFS as "new onset of persistent or relapsing, debilitating fatigue lasting at least six months in a person with no previous history of similar symptoms." The condition usually sets in after a heavy cold or bout of flu.

Many experts believe that CFS strikes when the body's immune system malfunctions and produces too many killer cells. Exhaustion, weakness, depression, and muscle and joint pain are all thought to be side effects of killer cell action.

CFS is a highly controversial disease. There are many who believe it is "all in the mind." Others passionately deny that this is the case. There seems so far to be no way to effectively treat it. Doctors recommend complete rest and stress reduction, but some experts are coming around to the idea that the disorder is related to hormonal imbalance.

Hormones and Depression

In his book, *The Good News about Depression* (1995), Dr. Mark

Gold points out that women are more likely to experience depression during their perimenopausal years (before menopause), when ovarian hormones are fluctuating, than after menopause, when they stabilize again. Gold sees a link between depression and estrogen's effect on serotonin levels. Low serotonin levels are associated with depression. Gold ponders whether estrogen therapy might work as a treatment for depression.

Many experts, including Elizabeth Lee Vliet, author of *Screaming to Be Heard*, and Dr. James Alexander Hamilton, author of *Postpartum Psychiatric Illness: A Picture Puzzle* (1992), have explored the effect of hormones on the brain and how they influence our mood, our sexuality, and symptoms normally associated with aging. Estrogen is just one of those hormones. If estrogen therapy can alleviate depression in women, perhaps it might be a better choice than Prozac?

And to take this argument one step further, if hormonal therapy or balancing your hormones through diet, exercise, and stress reduction can make a woman feel more energetic and vital, perhaps it might be a better choice than expensive antiaging creams, drugs, and surgery.

Hormonal Therapy in the 30s

Don't automatically assume if you get symptoms of hormonal imbalance that you are heading for perimenopause. Feeling out of shape, tired, and anxious can have as much to do with our lifestyle as with our hormones. More often than not in our 30s all that is needed to ease the symptoms is a change in diet and lifestyle to get us back on track. It should be pointed out, though, that in some cases no amount of diet, exercise, or stress reduction can reduce the symptoms, and hormonal therapy is necessary.

Imbalances of sex, stress, and blood sugar hormones in your 30s can destroy the quality of your life. Weight gain, fatigue, and bloating can slow you down. Infertility can be devastating. Irregular or heavy, painful periods make you feel uncomfortable. Acne is irritating. Facial hair is embarrassing. Mood swings and depression can stop you in your tracks. Anything that destroys the quality of your life deserves medical attention. If your hormones are in a state of imbalance, your body is in a state of crisis. The endocrine system revolves around a complex system of checks, balances, and interrelationships. Problems with one gland are eventually going to affect other glands and then affect your whole body. Your health will suffer.

Since the 1950s millions of women have been treated with hormones by their doctors. These hormones modify our biological functions or attempt to correct hormonal deficiency or excess. Many of us, despite the proven success record of hormonal therapy, are still reluctant to undergo treatment. We want to explore other alternatives. Our doctors, however, often don't consider what our preferences are. Hormonal therapy works, so hormonal therapy is prescribed.

Fear of side effects is the usual complaint when hormonal therapy is advised. We are correct to be concerned here. Each form of hormonal therapy carries with it certain risks. The pill is most often prescribed for women in their 30s with symptoms of hormonal imbalance, but it can cause nausea, possible weight gain, and mood swings. It also totally abolishes the normal menstrual cycle, distorts metabolism, and may cause blood clots, infertility, and birth defects. Another drawback of hormonal therapy is that it is not temporary. It becomes a part of your life. The casual prescription of hormones for women is certainly to be deplored. It is all too often used by doctors as a quick fix when simple lifestyle changes might be equally effective.

The term hormonal therapy carries with it the implication of a disease that needs to be treated. But perimenopause and menopause are not diseases. They are a natural state for your body to be in. If your doctor is advising hormonal therapy for these conditions you should certainly have your reservations and consider all options, including safer alternatives, before you make your decision.

However, a hormonal disorder in your 30s that is not due to symptoms of perimenopause is not a natural state for your body to be in. There is a strong case for arguing that it does merit hormonal therapy. Sure there are risks attached, but the benefits often outweigh the risks. Changes in diet and lifestyle have been shown to have the potential to change the course of hormonal imbalance, but in some cases, such as severe PCOS for instance, hormonal therapy from your doctor is still the only proven therapy. Whatever you decide, bear in mind that even if you are prescribed hormonal therapy, which is often the pill, your doctor should strongly recommend that you cultivate a healthy lifestyle to complement your treatment.

Alternatives to Hormonal Therapy

If you are experiencing hormonal imbalances but are not sure if you want to take synthetic hormones, there are natural options available. Pro-Gest is a natural progesterone hormone cream recommended for women with irregular or absent periods and hair loss. For women with fluctuating estrogen levels, mild plant estrogens—phytoestrogens—can help. Natural hormones will be discussed in greater detail in the next chapter dealing with perimenopause.

Other women find relief from alternative therapies, such as Chinese medicine, nutritional therapy, and aromatherapy, which are becoming increasingly popular alternatives to conventional treatments.

Other Hormonal Conditions

We've looked in depth at imbalances of the sex hormones, but other types of imbalances can occur in our 30s.

An overactive thyroid gland (hyperthyroidism) is most common in the 20 to 40 age range. Women are far more likely to suffer from it than men. Stress, smoking, genetics, and the use of certain medications are associated with this disorder. Like other common hormonal disorders, it's easy to overlook problems with the thyroid gland because the symptoms mimic many of the changes we associate with aging.

Hyperthyroidism occurs when the thyroid gland pumps out too much of its hormones. The excess hormones push the body's metabolism too hard, producing symptoms like rapid heartbeat, weight loss, nervousness, and weakness. Autoimmune disorders like Grave's disease can cause hyperthyroidism. Rapid weight loss and bulging eyes are a common symptom of Grave's disease. Drugs can usually be prescribed to balance hormonal production from the thyroid, and failing that, surgery may be necessary.

Hypothyroidism is the opposite of hyperthyroidism. It is unlikely, but it can occur in the 30s. It slows down the body's metabolism making weight gain more likely. Fatigue, chills, dry skin, heavy periods, swelling and puffiness around the face and eyes are but a few of the symptoms of hypothyroidism. It can also affect mental function and cause forgetfulness and depression. Sex drive and fertility can also be affected. The condition can be treated by giving sluggish thyroid glands pills which can restore the balance of the thyroid gland. The only drawback is that they have to be taken for life.

Problems with the thyroid gland can be detected with a simple blood test, and although symptoms can be alleviated with stress reduction and a healthy lifestyle, more often than not the only remedy is through hormonal therapy.

Imbalances of stress and blood sugar hormones, because they affect sex hormones, can have symptoms similar to imbalances of sex hormone. And because the hormonal systems are all interconnected, sooner or later if the imbalance is not corrected, the sex hormones will be affected anyway, producing symptoms associated with perimenopause.

Blood sugar hormones regulate the amount of sugar we have in our blood. Stress hormones help us cope with the stresses and strains of everyday life. Imbalances occur when diet is poor or when there is too much stress. For example, symptoms like depression, mood swings, and even weight gain have a lot to do with your diet. If you eat a diet high in processed carbohydrates and sugar, a flood of sugar is released into the bloodstream. The pancreas responds to the blood sugar imbalance by secreting the hormone insulin, which restores the blood sugar balance. But if diet continues to be high in sugar the body becomes progressively less sensitive to insulin. Diabetes, weight gain, and mood swings are possible results.

Similarly, if you are under too much stress the adrenal glands go into overdrive. Stress hormone is pumped into the blood. If the stress continues this can have long-term health effects on the balance of sex hormones and cause symptoms like irregular periods, acne, and infertility.

Stress reduction, regular exercise, and a healthy diet are often all that are needed to correct imbalances of stress and blood sugar hormones. Many women are surprised to find that symptoms such as fatigue, weight gain, and mood swings all but disappear when simple adjustments are made to lifestyle and diet.

There is so much we still don't understand about hormones, how they function and how imbalances can affect us. We do know, however, that in our 30s our hormone levels are not as stable as they were in our 20s. They begin to fluctuate, making us much more vulnerable to symptoms of hormonal imbalance. But we also know that a poor diet, lack of exercise, and too much stress can all contribute to hormonal problems. Part Three of this book shows how simple lifestyle changes can reduce the risk of hormonal problems and maximize our chances of health and vitality.

Chapter 7
Perimenopause

"Sounds cute, doesn't it, the peri-meni, but don't be fooled. This five to ten years preshutdown is when you feel most loopy" (Spillane and McKee, p. 160).

"Hot flashes, painful sex. I thought I wouldn't have to deal with this until I was at least fifty." (Michelle, age 35)

Even though there are around 40 million women in America who are at present experiencing perimenopause, little is known about the condition because it is a new area of research. But interest is growing. Women of our generation want to know what is happening to their bodies and how they can help themselves. We aren't content to sit on the sidelines anymore and blindly accept all that the doctors tell us. We want to understand our hormones and what we can do to help if there are problems.

The medical profession is beginning to take note. Progress is slow, but it is being made. Since the early 1990s the Association of Reproductive Health Professionals has held a series of conferences about perimenopause which highlight the latest research. It took a while for the medical establishment to take the symptoms of menopause seriously and confirm that they were not "all in the mind." So it will probably take a while before all doctors take symptoms of perimenopause seriously, despite that fact that many women know instinctively when something doesn't feel right.

"Over the past six months," says Anna, "I have become noticeably more irritable and short tempered. I'm not sleeping well either. I'm thirty-five, still menstruating, and I'm not having hot flashes so I can't be in menopause. My doctor tells me not to worry but I feel as if something is going on."

Peri-What?

Perimenopause is the period of 5 to 10 years before menstruation stops, when we experience declining, fluctuating sex hormone levels. It's impossible to be precise about the age you will reach perimenopause. All that can be said is that it usually occurs between the ages of 35 and 50, but it can happen earlier.

Certain factors could well influence how early you enter perimenopause. These include: heredity, the age that your mother went through it, smoking, being a vegetarian, very low cholesterol levels, eating disorders, being underweight, being overweight, not having children, African-American origin, Mediterranean or Southern European origin, lower socioeconomic background, pituitary gland problems, and ovaries that have been medically irradiated.

How long perimenopause lasts, how a woman feels, and what she experiences has a lot to do with hormones and genes but also a lot to do with her lifestyle, nutrition, activity levels, stress levels, and other factors. The process is different for every woman and involves far more than disruption to the normal menstrual cycle. It can affect the whole body.

Until recently doctors only thought of sex hormones in terms of the reproductive cycle and sexual organs, but research has discovered that there are actually sex hormone receptors in almost all the cells of the body. Estrogen, progesterone, and androgen are not just sex hormones with the purpose of giving us our sexual characteristics, our periods and, if we want, babies. There are estrogen receptors on brain cells, progesterone receptors on bones, receptors for both on white cells, and nearly everywhere else. Research has shown that maintaining estrogen levels can prevent senility after menopause. Progesterone can prevent our bones from thinning.

Androgen strengthens our muscles. Marked decline of these hormones can lead to mental confusion and osteoporosis, and can generally accelerate the process of aging in nearly every part of a woman's body.

It is not only after menopause, when hormone levels decline, that we should be concerned. In the years preceding menopause, levels of estrogen, progesterone, and androgen gradually begin to decline. Declining levels of hormones in the period now known as perimenopause will affect how a woman thinks, feels, and acts.

What Are the Symptoms?

Perhaps you haven't felt too well lately and you are not sure why. You think it might have something to do with your hormones. But if you went to a doctor, although you might be given a symptom relieving drug, more often than not you will be told that it is just your age and that there is nothing to worry about.

Perimenopause is not a disease. It is a natural stage for the body to be in, so in a sense, your doctor is right. In the words of nutritionist Ann Gittleman in her excellent manual on perimenopause *Before the Change*, "Perimenopause should not be thought of as a disease or treated like one. It is a naturally occurring transition before the change" (1999, p. 7). But just like menopause it is a time in our lives when we shouldn't have to suffer because our hormones are adjusting. Doctors need to take our complaints more seriously.

Here, listed as comprehensibly as possible, are the symptoms of perimenopause. None of them are pleasant and most of them can make you feel that your youthful energy and resilience are slipping away.

- Skin problems like acne, dry skin, wrinkles, and age spots
- Dark circles under the eyes
- Headaches, migraines, nausea

- Dizziness
- Feeling irritable
- Swollen ankles and feet
- Low blood sugar, trembling
- Anxiety
- Aches and pains
- Bloating
- Blood sugar imbalance
- Bone loss
- Breast changes
- Depression
- Male hair growth
- Fatigue
- Hair loss or thinning
- Hot flashes
- Insomnia
- Leg cramps
- Low noise tolerance
- Irregular periods
- Markedly worse PMS
- Muddled thinking
- Mood swings
- Muscular weakness
- Night sweats
- Panic attacks
- Loss of interest in sex
- Sleep disturbances
- Stomach cramps
- Teeth troubles
- Incontinence
- Vaginal dryness
- Urinary infections
- Water retention
- Weight gain and inability to lose it
- Weeping

This is not to say that all these symptoms will occur. No two women are the same, and each will have a different experience of perimenopause. Some of us may get insomnia, weight gain, and irregular periods, while others get the irregular periods and the mood swings but not the insomnia. Some of us may suffer greatly, others will barely notice any problems.

How Do I Know If I'm in Perimenopause?

Symptoms of perimenopause can be bewildering. You may feel that you really don't have much control over how you feel and, at times, how you look.

Sometimes it can be hard to recognize what exactly is going on, because perimenopausal symptoms are often similar to symptoms of PMS. In *Before the Change* Gittleman tells us how we can distinguish between symptoms of perimenopause and PMS. "If your period continues to be regular it's PMS. If your periods are irregular its perimenopause" (p. 7).

If you are in your mid-to-late 30s and you notice a pattern of continuing menstrual irregularity, the chances are you are entering perimenopause. In the early stages, hormonal therapy may not be as necessary as additional nutrients, regular exercise, creams, and natural hormonal therapy. It may, however, be necessary in the later stages.

It is possible to alleviate many of the symptoms through lifestyle changes. Women who wish to avoid drug therapy can manage symptoms of perimenopause. Depending on how far along you are in perimenopause, it may be possible to avoid drug therapy altogether (see "Dealing with Perimenopause").

If periods are regular but you notice that you have other symptoms like depression, bloating, and so on, you are probably not entering perimenopause yet. You may find that symptoms disappear with a simple change in diet and lifestyle as discussed later in this chapter. It is important also to stress at this point that in some cases irregular periods and symptoms resembling perimenopause may not indicate perimenopause at all but some other form of hormonal imbalance, like androgen disorder or problems with the thyroid gland. That's why it's vital you don't assume automatically that you are in perimenopause if you get irregular periods and that you go and see your doctor to find out what exactly is causing the problem.

Early Menopause

There is a strong likelihood that some of us will experience perimenopausal symptoms in our 30s, while menopause at this time in our lives is less likely. However, there are cases when menopause strikes unusually early. "Since 7 to 11 percent of women go through premature menopause before age forty, according to Dr. Richard Bronson, physicians should not tell women they won't go through menopause until they are about fifty" (Ford, p. 44).

Women in their 30s with symptoms of menopause like hot flashes, depression, and gradual ovarian failure are not being treated seriously by their doctors. Doctors still assume that the 30s are far too young for a woman to go through menopause. But there are too many exceptions now for this to be a justifiable response. Women who are not given hormonal therapy but other kinds of drugs or counseling are not being treated appropriately.

During menopause, the ovaries make fewer and fewer hormones. Cycles become irregular because ovulation cannot take place and eventually they cease altogether. A woman's reproductive life is over unless scientific and medical manipulation is resorted to. Pregnancy is now possible after menopause using donor eggs from other women, but it is very unlikely. Other symptoms that accompany menopause include night sweats, panic attacks, mood swings, reduction in breast size, loss of libido, bone thinning, and weight gain.

Early menopause can come as a great shock to younger women in our ageist culture. There is the fear that as soon as women go through menopause their bodies will simply fall apart and waste away without medication, particularly hormones. Aging is associated with decline, even though decline is not a natural consequence of aging. We fear menopause and in our minds associate it with neurotic old women with hot flashes and foul tempers. As a result, many women who go through early menopause expect their bodies to deteriorate, when this is not the case at all.

The idea that menopause means getting old and no longer having a role to fulfill in society is obsolete due to changes in cultural standards and advances in medical research. Today a woman's importance is no longer measured and defined in terms of the use she makes of her reproductive organs, and just because she cannot bear children does not mean she cannot be sexual. Modern research has shown that many of the uncomfortable feelings that accompany menopause are not due to decline, atrophy, or decay, but to hormonal change. The common physical discomforts of menopause result from a lack of progesterone, estrogen, and androgen. Hormonal therapy can be sought to ease these discomforts. And more and more is also being discovered about how proper diet, exercise, and alternative therapies can alleviate the symptoms of both perimenopause and menopause for those who want to avoid hormonal therapy.

If menopause does happen to you in your 30s, your attitude will be important to the bodily change taking place. If you see it not as a sign of aging and decline but as a hormonal change taking place in your body, you can discover that menopause is a positive experience. It brings dramatic and often difficult changes. As Joan Borysenko writes in her insightful study *A Woman's Book of Life*, menopause can be seen as a "second puberty, an initiation into what is the most powerful, exciting and fulfilling" part of a woman's life (p. 140). We can find fulfillment both personally and socially. In freeing us from the reproductive cycle, this stage in life offers us the opportunity to fully understand ourselves, our sexuality, and what we have to contribute to the world.

Dealing with Perimenopause

Many of the symptoms of perimenopause can be alleviated through balanced diet, getting the right amount of exercise, and stress reduction. A balanced diet with enough carbohydrates, protein, and fat will help regulate fluctuating hormone levels (although advocates of low-fat diets or high protein diets or high carbohydrate diets for health and weight loss don't really take this into account).

Low- or no-fat diets are very hard to stay on for any length of time and often end in binge eating, and they don't give the body enough of the good fats it needs to manufacture hormones. Basically, too little fat in your diet can make symptoms of hormonal imbalance worse. With insufficient amounts of essential nutrients, symptoms will not go away.

For balancing your hormones a healthy diet is crucial. Unhealthy eating often produces symptoms undistinguishable from peri-menopausal symptoms. If you have been suffering you may find that simple changes in diet will alleviate the symptoms completely. We will discuss diet in detail in Chapter 8.

Alongside changes in diet, exercise and stress reduction can also help alleviate the symptoms of perimenopause. Moderate exercise helps all the hormone systems function better. It is now widely recognized that exercise evokes hormonal responses from the body. Aerobic exercise reduces your insulin level and elevates glucagon. Anaerobic exercise causes the body to secrete human growth hormone, which is a great fat burner. Glucagon promotes circulation.

Exercise can combat depression or stress because it releases endorphins, neurotransmitters that heighten mood. Exercise helps weight control, lessens the risk of osteoporosis, and helps raise metabolism and the absorption of nutrients. Exercise can help just about every symptom of perimenopause.

Reducing the amount of stress in your life will also alleviate symptoms of hormonal imbalance. Stress levels are controlled by the adrenal hormones. If stress is constant, an excessive amount of stress hormone will be produced and this can lead to diabetes, high blood pressure, depression, and hormonal imbalance. The adrenals will eventually become exhausted and not supply enough sex hormones in the amount needed, with consequent symptoms.

The adrenal gland can be rejuvenated through stress reduction and making sure your diet includes sufficient amounts of vitamin B_5; other B vitamins, especially B_2 and B_{12}; vitamin C; vitamin E; zinc; and manganese.

Eating a regulated diet, exercising regularly, and managing stress can often alleviate symptoms of perimenopause experienced by women in their 30s and 40s. Avoiding food and water contaminants as much as possible will help too, as these can unsettle the hormonal balance in your body.

Although the onset of perimenopause may cause anxiety and the feeling that "I'm too young for this," don't let it overwhelm you. Remember that perimenopause is not a disease but a natural state when your body experiences hormonal changes as it prepares for menopause that usually happens in the 50s. Sometimes, though, self-help measures, stress reduction, diet, and exercise alone may not be enough. You may need to resort to some kind of hormone therapy.

Most of us will have heard about the benefits and risks of hormone replacement therapy. We probably have an opinion about it already. We still know so little about hormones and the effects of hormone replacement therapy, and more and more experts are coming to the conclusion that perhaps a more natural approach to balancing our hormones is the answer. A lot of us are not aware of natural options to synthetic hormones, so we'll begin with them.

Natural Hormones

If your periods are irregular and you are having a lot of anovulatory cycles, you probably are not producing enough progesterone. As well as preparing the body for pregnancy, progesterone helps burn fat; stabilizes uterine lining growth; helps prevent breast cancer, heart disease, and bone loss; stabilizes blood sugar balance; and acts as an antidepressant. It also counteracts the undesirable effects of estrogen dominance, which include bloating, depression, weight gain, breast swelling, irregular periods, sugar craving, loss of sex drive, tiredness, and water retention.

If perimenopausal symptoms do not disappear through diet and exercise alone, it might be worth trying a natural progesterone cream. Apply the cream daily as often as you like in different areas of the skin such as the upper chest, inner arms, backs of hands and breasts. It may take several weeks for the progesterone to take its effect in the tissues. Try to find a cream that includes more than 400 milligrams per ounce. Recommended creams included Pro-Gest, Angel Care, and Pro-Alo. You can order them by mail from Uni-Key Health Systems (800-888-4353) if you can't find them in a health-food store. You may also prefer to take natural progesterone as an oral capsule.

Fluctuating estrogen levels at perimenopause can also cause discomfort. To alleviate these symptoms we can take mild plant estrogens called phytoestrogen. Phytoestrogens are found in plant foods such as soybean, and herbs such as dong quai and black cohosh, which can stimulate the body's estrogen production if levels are low and lower levels that are too high. Foods rich in phytoestrogens include soy, apples, asparagus, carrots, beans, cereals, corn, garlic, legumes, milk, oats, olive oil, pears, peas, rice bran, rye, dried sea vegetables, sweet potato, and wheat germ.

Synthetic Hormones

If you are suffering from perimenopausal symptoms and consult a doctor of conventional medicine, the chances are you will be placed on synthetic hormones. If you have vaginal dryness and hot flashes, for example, you will probably be prescribed Premarin or estrogen replacement. If you are not menstruating and suffer from bloating you will probably be given Provera or progesterone replacement.

Provera and Premarin do act as quick fixes. Symptoms may disappear and many women I spoke to said they felt great. Others, however, said that they didn't feel right on synthetic hormone replacement therapy.

Premarin and Provera are not identical to a woman's natural hormones. There are also severe health risks attached to overmedication with Premarin and Provera. These include blood clots, breast cancer, breast tenderness, depression, fatigue, gallstones, hair loss, headaches, nausea, loss of sexual desire, uterine cancer, weight gain, and yeast infection.

Provera, Premarin, and the birth control pill all have unpleasant side effects but these side effects vary from woman to woman. What works for one woman won't work for another. We all have different hormone levels, different metabolic rates, different bodies, and different personalities. What is a normal hormone level for one woman may be abnormal for another. You have to find what works best for you.

Androgen Disorders

Perimenopausal symptoms can often be confused with symptoms of androgen disorder, which tends to strike women in their 30s. Androgen disorder occurs when too much testosterone, or so-called male hormones, is produced by the ovaries and adrenal gland. Symptoms include irregular periods, weight gain, male hair growth, acne, thinning hair, dry skin, infertility, and metabolic problems that increase the risk of diabetes and heart disease. Symptoms of androgen disorder often need hormonal therapy, but they can be relieved if attention is paid to diet, exercise, stress reduction, and weight management. Supplementing with nutrients that boost an exhausted adrenal gland—like vitamins B, C, zinc, and manganese—will certainly help too.

The most usual treatment offered by doctors for androgen excess is the pill, which decreases androgen levels but also contains estrogen and progesterone, or if you cannot take the pill, Gn-RH analogues and estrogen replacement. For women with symptoms of excessive androgens—for example, male hair growth and acne—but normal androgen levels, another set of treatments can block the effect of androgens on skin and hair and these are called androgen antagonists. The drug most commonly used in the United States is called Spironoclactone.

Nonhormonal treatments offered by doctors for androgen problems include retinoids (a form of vitamin A) and antibiotics. Androgen excess is far more common in your 30s than androgen deficiency. Sometimes, though, symptoms of androgen deficiency will occur during perimenopause; these include loss of interest in sex, loss of muscle tone, thinning hair, and irregular periods. You might consider natural testosterone creams or testosterone replacement therapy.

If you wish to conceive and have high androgen levels or a

problem with estrogen and progesterone levels, all of which can suppress ovulation, fertility drugs will be used to induce ovulation.

Testing Your Hormone Levels

If you want to find out about your estrogen, progesterone, and androgen levels, hormone tests can give you an indication of whether your hormones are in balance or not. Bear in mind, though, that hormone levels fluctuate on various days of your cycle. Time of day can also be a factor to consider. Blood tests and urine tests are the kinds most readily available from your doctor, but it is possible to do your own saliva test at home.

Saliva tests are particularly accurate for testing progesterone levels. For more information contact Aeron Lifecycles in California (800-631-7900). Aeron will supply you with materials for saliva collection and mailing. The cost is around $50 per test, and you usually get results back in two weeks. Aeron makes it clear that its direct-to-consumer tests are meant only to monitor changes in hormonal levels. If you find the results hard to interpret see your doctor.

Experiencing perimenopausal symptoms can often be confusing and alarming. You may or may not go through perimenopause in your 30s, but if you do hopefully this section will have shown you that it is not to be feared. To repeat, it is a natural state for your body to be in, not a symptom of decline, and if you experience discomfort there are ways to reduce it. It is possible to go through the challenge of perimenopause and to enjoy your life at the same time.

The 30s are a decade of challenge. Perimenopause is just one of the many you may face. Understanding and managing your perimenopause can increase your levels of self-knowledge and self-acceptance. Part Three, which focuses more generally on improving all aspects of your health in your 30s, shows how the many other challenges you may face can also bring with them the maturity, confidence, and increased body awareness to help you look and feel better than ever before.

PART THREE
HEALTHY LIVING IN THE 30S

"*Age is a question of mind over matter. If you don't mind, it doesn't matter.*"

—Satchel Paige

•   •   •

"*It is much cheaper and more effective to maintain good health than it is to regain it once it is lost.*"

—Kenneth Cooper

Chapter 8
A Youthful Diet

When I started to come to terms with the fact that I wasn't truly young anymore, what gave me confidence was knowing that I could still look good. I had grown up seeing women mature with beauty, confidence, and style. These women had obviously taken care of themselves.

Time and time again women who are growing older with vitality and beauty told me that good looks in later life had nothing to do with antiaging creams or surgery. They were about a healthy diet, regular exercise, enjoying life, taking care of yourself, preparing for the bodily changes age brings, and avoiding what really takes its toll on your looks: junk food, hard living, stress, sun, and wind.

Not one of these women, however, claimed that such measures would prevent the gradual loss of youth. Obsession with appearance and with looking young will often have the opposite effect and make you look far older. You can look younger with a healthy diet, regular exercise, and a youthful outlook but not if these are carried to obsessive extremes. If looking young becomes the main focus of your life, the obsession has become unhealthy and aging. Women who continue to compare how they look with how they looked at eighteen won't ever be confident with their looks. No amount of moisturizer will give us our youth back.

Lived-in faces can have a glamour and a confidence that youth just can't match. Continuing good looks and attractiveness does not mean trying to preserve a twentysomething face and body. It means looking good at your age, not for your age. Trying to look like you did ten years ago is backward-looking and aging. Focusing on the present and looking forward in anticipation to the future is vitalizing and youthful.

The self-help tips in the chapters to follow won't show you how to turn back the clock, but they will show you how to prevent unnecessary aging damage and how to enhance what is lovely and unique about you. Let's start with the foundation stone of looking and feeling youthful: a balanced diet.

Eating Like a Grownup

If you want to look good, you have to start eating well. Few of us really realize that what we put in our mouths and stomachs may actually make us appear older than we are. Healthy eating habits almost certainly have a positive effect on our appearance. If we want to look vital and attractive in our 30s, it is time to mature beyond crash dieting and to cultivate a sensible eating plan for the rest of your life.

Understanding the basics of good nutrition can help us look and feel more youthful. In our 30s it is time to start eating like a grownup. Deficiencies in certain essential nutrients can accelerate normal aging processes, such as the immune system weakening or fatty deposits in the bloodstream or bones thinning. You can't get away with a diet of hot dogs and ice cream anymore. Your body lacks the resilience to support organs and systems when insufficient nutrients are taken in. Even those who are overweight could still be malnourished. The *Vogue* beauty experts describe this as a state of "affluent malnutrition" when even the best fed are undernourished (Hutton, p. 228). It is the quality of your diet, not the quantity of what you eat that matters. And a quality diet is a balanced diet.

A balanced diet contains all the nutrients you need to fight those processes that can accelerate aging. It will contain as wide a variety of foods as possible eaten in moderation. That means it may even include those foods traditionally thought to be unhealthy. For instance, recent research is showing that even the great "baddie," chocolate, is thought to contain antioxidants that fight aging. This

doesn't mean you should eat chocolate to excess. It just means that it can, like almost every other food, be eaten in moderation as part of a balanced diet.

One of the many benefits of a balanced diet is that it regulates blood sugar levels. Getting blood sugar levels back in balance is important for alleviating symptoms resembling perimenopause. Depression, mood swings, and even weight gain have as much to do with what you eat as with your hormone levels.

Depression and mood swings have been linked to low blood sugar levels. Low blood sugar levels stress the body because sugar (glucose) is the body's fuel. Messages are sent to the brain to find more sugar and that's why we start craving sweet things. Unfortunately, many of the foods we choose to satisfy these cravings, like doughnuts and chocolate bars, make the problem worse, causing even more blood sugar ups and downs.

It is conceivable that the high-carbohydrate, low-fat diet many thirtysomething women favor causes many of the symptoms of perimenopause. Low fat is considered to be the healthy way to eat in our society, despite the fact that since the beginning of the low-fat craze the health of Americans has not improved and obesity is on the increase. We believe that low fat can lower cholesterol levels, decrease the risk of heart disease, and stop us from getting fat. The problem is, though, that those of us on a low-fat diet tend to get food cravings and eat large amounts of carbohydrates like bread, fat-free cookies, and so on. By so doing, we elevate our blood sugar levels and our insulin levels and develop a condition known as "insulin resistance," when our body doesn't respond to insulin anymore (insulin is the hormone which regulates our blood sugar levels). We get moody and irritable. We put on weight.

If our diets are balanced it is highly likely that blood sugar levels will stabilize. Energy levels, concentration, and mood should improve. We will feel years younger. For stable blood sugar levels, hormonal regulation, and sustained physical and mental effort, a balanced diet

that contains all the nutrients we need is the sensible option.

Nutrients

Nutrients are substances in food that help us grow, repair, and sustain ourselves. If we haven't got them, we are likely to look and feel old and frail.

The nutrients we eat are our body's fuel. The right kind of fuel includes all six classes of nutrients in our diet: carbohydrates, proteins, fats, vitamins, minerals, and water. Carbohydrates, proteins, and fats are used by your body as a source of energy. Your body does not get energy from vitamins and minerals, but they are essential because they help various bodily processes and chemical reactions. For instance, magnesium is an important player in the process of releasing energy from the food we eat. Finally, water is the medium in which all your bodily reactions take place. Water makes up about 60 percent of our body, and without water we could not live.

If you take a good long look at yourself in the mirror from time to time you can tell a lot about your health and whether or not you are getting your nutrients. Malnutrition makes you look older than you are. Rings around the irises could indicate high cholesterol. Dark circles under the eyes could indicate circulatory problems.

Despite increased awareness of how important diet is to our well-being, a surprising number of women in their 30s only have a vague idea about what healthy eating is. We aren't that sure about the basics of good nutrition. What nutrients are essential for our well-being? What nutrients can keep us looking and feeling young?

Knowing what foods contain which nutrients, what is important for a diet that regulates your hormones, and what foods can make you feel vital and healthy will help you plan a balanced diet that includes a wide variety of foods, composed of a balance of carbohydrates, proteins, and fats that include the correct amount of vitamins, minerals, and water. Stable blood sugar is a great benefit

of a balanced diet. When blood sugar levels are normal, you will have more energy, be able to concentrate better, and feel more relaxed and happy. You are also less likely to have hormonal problems and to feel older than you are.

Proteins

Proteins are the substances that build tissues for growth and repair. When eaten, proteins are broken down into amino acids for use all over the body. We can't store proteins, so we need a constant supply. Amino acids are the building blocks of life because we use them to rebuild and repair our tissues and organs. Your skin, your hair, your muscles, and your hormones are all composed of proteins our bodies use.

If you don't get enough daily protein in your diet, your body will break down its own muscle tissue, and metabolism slows down. The result is loss of muscle tone, thinning hair, irritability, and fatigue, all of which are aging. Proteins also stabilize blood sugar levels by stimulating glucagon, which restores blood sugar levels and releases fat. Increased amounts of protein will increase your metabolic rate significantly, help burn fat, and give you more energy.

Proteins are found in foods like lean meat, seafood, cottage cheese, poultry, fowl, fish, eggs, milk and milk products, beans, nuts, yeast, soy, and wheat germ. Protein should account for about 25 to 30 percent of a balanced diet.

Carbohydrates

It is very important to eat the right kinds and amounts of carbohydrates in a balanced antiaging diet. Many experts believe that people who live on a low-fat diet and have symptoms like low energy, fatigue, mood swings, weight gain, dry skin, and dry hair have over-emphasized carbohydrates in their diet. They are deficient in hormone-balancing essential fatty acids that we get in dietary fat

and metabolic-raising protein.

All carbohydrates we eat are converted into blood sugar in the form of glucose. What our body doesn't need as fuel is stored as body fat, which is under the control of insulin. If we eat too many carbohydrates our blood sugar levels and our insulin levels rise. So if you have been eating a low-fat diet and still putting on weight perhaps high carbohydrate levels are to blame.

Carbohydrates are of two kinds, simple and complex. Simple carbohydrates are absorbed by the body quickly. They provide a rush of sugar and a fast insulin response. If too much sugar is consumed the pancreas can't produce enough insulin to keep up. "Late onset" diabetes may occur.

Diabetes tends to strike those who are overweight and sedentary. It is aging because it weakens our defenses against heart disease, encourages weight gain, and has many unpleasant side effects like dizziness and poor vision, sores on the arms and legs, and vaginal infections. Women in the 30s most at risk are those who are overweight or have a family history of diabetes. To reduce the risk of diabetes make sure you don't have an excessive intake of sugar and you exercise regularly and eat sensibly.

Complex carbohydrates take more time to be absorbed into the blood stream than simple sugars and are much better for us. Obviously, the faster food turns into a sugar the more undesirable it is. The glycemic index often used by diabetics lists foods according to how rapidly they induce insulin. Generally, simple sugars, processed carbohydrates, white flour, pasta, white rice or potatoes, corn chips or biscuits and cakes are high on the list. With complex carbohydrates, potatoes, oatmeal, peas, fruit and food high in fiber, like vegetables, fall low on the list.

Starch is a good source of carbohydrates, and it is found in bread, potatoes, rice, pasta, fruit, vegetables, and cereals. Sucrose (table sugar) is not a good source of carbohydrates, but natural sugars found in fruits and vegetables are fine. Fiber provides little energy but it is very important because it plays an important part in regular bowel

movements. Good sources are wholemeal bread and pasta, vegetables, and fruit. Opinions differ, but many nutritionists think that foods containing starch and fiber should make up about 40 to 50 percent of your diet, and perhaps not the 70 percent often recommended.

Fat

There is no doubt that a very high-fat diet is unhealthy. The more fat we consume, the more free radicals we are likely to ingest, and excess fat consumption has been linked to obesity, diabetes, heart disease, and certain types of cancer, particularly the breast and bowel. A high-fat diet can also increase the likelihood of gallstones developing. Gallstones develop when the gallbladder is worn out, as it has to cope with so much fat.

Watching our fat intake is important but, on the other hand, a diet that is too low in fat is prematurely aging. Many women in their 30s eat too little fat in the misguided belief that it will help them lose weight. But we need a certain amount of fat in our diet to burn and metabolize fat.

Dietary fats provide the essential fatty acids required to produce hormones. They assist in the absorption of vitamins and they nourish our skin and nerves and mucous membranes. They also signal to our brains that we have eaten enough. If enough fat has not been eaten we will still feel hungry.

Fats may be saturated or unsaturated. The difference is the combination of hydrogen atoms present in them. A simple test is that at room temperature saturated fats are solid and unsaturated are liquid. Unsaturated fats are further classified as polyunsaturated and monounsaturated, again referring to the bonds between the atoms they consist of. Most fats are a mixture of all the kinds of type, but one kind of fat predominates.

Fat in our diet enables our bodies to create eicosanoids, which are hormones that control bodily functions. Eicosanoids are vital for our health, well-being, and hormonal balance, and they are known to be affected by what we eat. For example, too many carbohydrates will increase eiconsanoids that work negatively to increase cholesterol and weaken immunity.

It is believed that if we eat too much saturated fat it can raise blood cholesterol to dangerous levels and increase our risk of cardiovascular problems and weight gain. Saturated fats are mainly of animal origin and are found in meat, milk, butter, cheese, soy oil, olive oil, and nuts. Polyunsaturated and monounsaturated fats have greater health benefits. They tend to occur in plants and they have lower blood cholesterol. Good sources are fish and seaweed, flaxseed oil, green leafy vegetables, liver, olive oil, and soy oil.

The jury is still out, but as far as a hormone-regulating diet is concerned, our diet should be about 20 to 30 percent fat with the emphasis on unsaturated fat.

Fatty Acids

According to Gittleman in *Before the Change*, many bodily functions and health benefits are associated with the metabolism of fatty acids and the eicosanoids fatty acids build (p. 60).

In our 30s, making sure we get enough fatty acids in our diet will relieve perimenopausal problems; lower the risk of blood clots; lower blood pressure; relieve migraines; boost libido; benefit skin, nails, and hair; encourage weight loss; combat depression; alleviate hangovers; check the spread of infection; and may even lower the risk of breast cancer. Without enough fatty acids, your body cannot manufacture stress and ovarian hormones. If your diet does not contain enough omega 3 and omega 6 fatty acid, health will suffer.

Omega 3 fatty acid can be found in the oils of cold water fish; certain vegetable, seed, and botanical oils are rich in omega 6 fatty acid. Our bodies cannot manufacture these fatty acids by themselves. Polyunsaturated fats tend to be high in omega fatty acids. These fatty acids control cell growth, lower cholesterol, distribute fat-soluble vitamins through body tissue, and are the building blocks for prostaglandins. Prostaglandins/eicosanoids are hormone-like substances that control our body functions. Prostaglandins are known to alleviate the symptoms of PMS and perimenopausal symptoms.

There are tremendous health benefits for women in their 30s associated with the metabolism of essential fatty acids and prostaglandins. They can certainly relieve symptoms of perimenopause. American women seem to be more deficient in omega 3 than in omega 6. A diet to regulate hormones needs to be not just sufficient but rich in both. Sources of omega 3 include seaweed, green leafy vegetables, and fresh coldwater fish. If you are not a fish eater you might consider taking fish oil capsules. Foods rich in omega 6 include green leafy vegetables, lean red meat, and flaxseed oil. Flaxseed oil is in fact high in both omega 3 as well as 6. Canola oil and soy oil are recommended too. Evening primrose oil and olive oil have also been shown to alleviate symptoms of perimenopause.

Vitamins and Minerals

To look your best your body needs the correct balance of vitamins and minerals. Deficiency in any vitamin or mineral can make you feel unwell. For example, if your diet is deficient in iron, symptoms include anemia, brittle hair, hair loss, difficulty swallowing, dizziness, fatigue, fragile bones, brittle nails, obesity, and slow reaction time. Lack of iron-rich foods, or iron-depleting foods such as caffeine which can rob the system of iron, heavy and prolonged menstruation, and intense exercise can all cause iron deficiency. Deficiency in potassium can lead to tiredness and depression.

Here's a brief look of the major vitamins and minerals every woman in her 30s should ensure her diet includes, with special emphasis on those that can alleviate perimenopausal symptoms.

Vitamin A fights infection and prevents dry skin and poor bone growth. It is found in vegetables, milk, butter, margarine, and egg yolks.

Thiamin is important for carbon dioxide removal during respiration.

It is found in whole grains, nuts, and seeds.

Riboflavin is needed for cell renewal and is found in milk, meat, eggs, and leafy vegetables.

Niacin helps to prevent disease, improve the mood, and promote a glowing complexion. You can find it in milk, eggs, cheeses, and fish.

Pantothenic acid is essential for energy metabolism and stress reduction. It is found in many foods such as meat, fish, poultry, whole grain cereals, and dried beans.

Vitamin B_6 is important for the metabolism of proteins. It can relieve water retention, bloating, skin problems, depression, and symptoms of perimenopause. It has the ability to boost progesterone levels and reduce estrogen levels. It is also needed for the normal secretion of serotonin, the brain neurotransmitter that regulates mood, sleep, and appetite. Vitamin B_6 is also important in collagen formation and bone strength. Women on the contraceptive pill must ensure that they get adequate vitamin B_6. Food sources include spinach, bananas, liver, nuts, meat, fish, legumes, and green peppers. Vitamin B_6 can be taken on its own, but the B vitamins are absorbed better if taken in complex form.

Vitamin B_{12} promotes healthy skin and helps maintain a healthy nervous system. It is found in meat, milk, eggs, cheese, and fish.

Biotin is important for carbohydrate and fat metabolism. It is found in liver, peanuts, and cheese.

Folate promotes cell production and healthy skin and is found in leafy green vegetables, chicken, liver, and kidneys.

Vitamin C, found in green vegetables and citrus fruits, prevents colds, heals wounds, and is essential for normal metabolism and the reduction of menstrual problems. It boosts the immune system, fights fatigue, and protects us from toxins.

Vitamin D, good for bone growth and calcium absorption, is also an aid in relieving menstrual problems and is found in tuna, eggs, butter, and cheese.

Vitamin E promotes blood clotting and is found in milk, vegetables, liver, rice, and bran. Diets low in fat are often deficient in vitamin E, which is essential for hormonal balance in women. Good food sources include vegetable oils, nuts, and seeds. Vitamin E can alleviate perimenopausal symptoms such as hot flashes and breast tenderness.

Vitamin K is active in maintaining the involuntary nervous system, vascular system, and involuntary muscles. It is found in wheat germ, vegetable oil, and whole grain bread and cereal.

Minerals

Calcium prevents blood clotting and is necessary for bone growth, healthy teeth, and iron absorption. It is found in milk and milk products, egg yolks, green vegetables, and shellfish. Calcium deficiency causes bone loss, as the milk ads constantly remind us. Most of us know that calcium deficiency is a health risk. What we probably don't know, however, is that most of us aren't calcium deficient, we simply lack the ability to utilize the calcium we have because we don't have enough magnesium in our diet. Calcium needs magnesium to be incorporated into your bones. If there is not enough magnesium the extra calcium will collect in soft tissues, not bones, and cause arthritis. Dairy products contain more calcium than magnesium.

Many women in their 30s have a calcium/magnesium imbalance because we avoid magnesium-rich food like almonds, nuts, seeds, and sea vegetables. Magnesium deficiency can cause perimenopausal symptoms. It has a sedative effect and symptoms include depression, nervousness, anxiety, concentration problems, frequent urination, increase in body odor, constipation, and fatigue.

Chromium normalizes insulin levels so that sugar can be processed more quickly. Foods rich in the mineral include brewer's yeast, liver, some shellfish, and mushrooms.

Copper is an aid in the metabolism of iron and is found in liver and whole grains.

Fluoride strengthens teeth and is found in fluorinated water and tea.

Iron is the basic component of blood hemoglobin and prevents anemia. If your diet is deficient in iron you will feel tired and lethargic and listless. You may also have pale skin, dark circles under the eyes, and feel the cold more. Irritability and headaches are also associated with iron deficiency. A lot of physical activity, pregnancy, and nursing can severely deplete iron amounts. As well as this, iron deficiency can cause eating disorders and interfere with thyroid function. On the other hand, too much iron is not ideal either. This can increase the risk of heart disease and cancer. Women who don't menstruate or who have stopped menstruating often have high levels of iron. Iron can be found in dark green leafy vegetable, beans, eggs, dried fruit, and liver. Iron intake increases if vitamin C intake increases. Red wine and dark beer also increase iron absorption. On the other hand caffeine, aspirin, and some food preservatives interfere with iron absorption.

Iodine is an aid in regulating energy use in the body. It is found in seaweed and seafood.

Magnesium, found in milk, grains, vegetables, fruits, and cereals, is involved in the normal functioning of the brain, spinal cord, and nerves, and is an aid in forming bones.

Potassium is needed for healthy nerves and muscles and is found in milk, vegetables, and fruit.

Sodium helps maintain adequate water in cells in the body and is found in table salt, milk, and meat.

Phosphorus, found in milk, yogurt, yeast, and wheat germ, is required for bone growth, strong teeth, and energy transformation.

Zinc plays an essential part in keeping the reproductive organs and the body's enzyme systems healthy. Zinc is also important for perimenopausal women because it is needed for bone formation. Zinc supplements can actually slow bone loss and boost the immune system. Women who are zinc deficient tend to have high copper levels. Low zinc and high copper levels will cause perimenopausal symptoms. Zinc deficiency is caused by stress and a high sugar, high carbohydrate diet. Certain medications can cause zinc deficiency, as can alcohol and high-fiber vegetarian diets. Food sources of zinc include red meat, egg yolk, milk, nuts, peas, beans, seafood, and whole grains. Vegetarians should ensure that they get sufficient zinc.

Figure 3 gives a list of the recommended dietary allowances adapted from the Food and Nutrition Board of the National Academy of Sciences. The recommended daily allowance (RDA) is, however, surprisingly controversial, and you will see it differ from expert to expert. As things stand now, the RDA prevents most nutrient deficiency diseases but many scientist believe they should be substantially increased to reflect the mounting evidence that larger does can delay the process of aging and prevent and treat many diseases.

The RDA is in the process of being replaced by new guidelines, the dietary reference intakes (DRI) issued by the Food and Nutrition Board which determines the RDA. Two RDAs have already been dramatically increased: calcium and folic acid. It is still not okay to take large doses of vitamin and mineral supplements though.

Figure 3

RDA for Vitamins and Minerals			
Nutrient	**RDA** (recommended daily allowance)	**Nutrient**	**RDA** (recommended daily allowance)
Vitamin A	800 mcg RE	Vitamin K	65 mcg
Vitamin B_1	1.1 mg	Calcium	800 mg
Vitamin B_2	1.3 mg	Iodine	150 mcg
Vitamin B_3	15 mg	Iron	15 mg
Vitamin B_6	1.6 mg	Magnesium	280 mg
Vitamin B_{12}	2.0 mcg	Phosphorus	800 mg
Folic acid	180 mcg	Selenium	55 mcg
Vitamin C	50 mg	Zinc	12 mg
Vitamin D	5 mcg	Protein	50 g
Vitamin E	8 mg		

RE=retinol equivalents, mg=milligrams, mcg=micrograms

How Much Should I Eat Each Day?

Food guides can not only help you assess the nutritional value of your diet but also help you determine if you are eating too much or to little. Remember though, these recommendations are not perfect, and as scientists discover new information, food guides change and nutritionists revise their opinions. A balanced diet should contain the right quantity of food for you. How much you need will depend on how active you are and what your build is. It may not be on the bestsellers list, but the U.S. Department of Agriculture Guide is a reliable reference for information on daily food intake, healthy eating, healthy living and healthy aging (see Figure 4).

Figure 4: The U.S. Department of Agriculture Food Pyramid

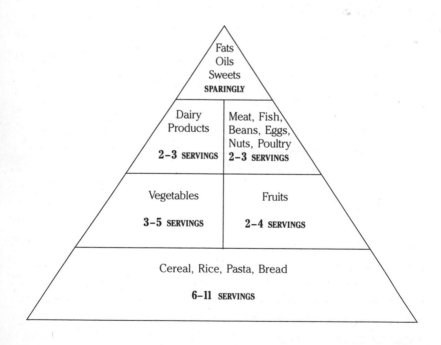

At present the bread, rice, cereal, and pasta food group recommendation is 6 to 11 servings a day (1 serving is a slice of bread) The fruit group is 2–4 servings a day. The vegetable group: 3–5 servings a day. The dairy products group: 2–3 servings a day (1 serving is 1 cup of milk or yogurt, 1 ounce of cheese, or 2 cups of cottage cheese). Meat, poultry, fish, eggs, and nuts are 2–3 servings a day (1 serving is 1 cup of beans, 3 ounces of meat or fish). Fats, oils, and sweets are to be eaten sparingly.

The U.S. Department of Agriculture Guide is helpful, but for women in their 30s, especially those experiencing perimenopausal symptoms, consideration should be given to a reduction in servings from the carbohydrate food group and a proportionate increase in hormone-regulating fat, according to the guidelines given previously.

An Antiaging Diet

In our 30s our metabolic needs decrease and the quantity of our food should also decrease. But although we should be cutting down on junk food, we should actually be eating more healthy food such as fruit, vegetables, fish, and whole grains. Every calorie we eat from our 30s onwards should be more nutritious than when we were in our 20s and could afford to eat more.

As research into the protective effect of food continues, it becomes clear that a diet that mimics that of our early hunting, fishing, and gathering ancestors is perhaps the healthiest. This is a diet that is lower in saturated fat and wheat intake than we have today, with much higher levels of vitamin C and calcium, not from dairy products, but from fruit and vegetables. A primitive diet of regular fresh fish, fruits, vegetables, nuts, and seeds may be able to beat many of the degenerative diseases suffered in the modern world. Recent guidelines for healthy eating recognize this. Recommendations from the World Health Organization include that fish be eaten as often as meat, that we eat at least five to nine servings of fruit and vegetables a day, and that we eat seeds and nuts and complex starchy carbohydrates with every meal.

Meat is a good source of vitamins, minerals, and protein, but it is high in saturated fat and eating it more than a few times a week isn't good for the health of the digestive system. Fish, on the other hand, has far more health benefits. It contains protein and a class of fatty acids essential to heart and brain function and hormone regulation. Oily fish seems to be protective against heart disease.

Cutting down on saturated fat isn't difficult if you just have unprocessed food instead of the packaged alternative. Cookies, cakes, chocolate, pastry, and potato chips contain vast amounts of saturated fat, as does processed meat, so it makes sense to switch to lean meat. Strangely, most of us are more concerned about our cholesterol levels than how much saturated fat we eat. Many women avoid eggs for that reason, but in the process they are depriving themselves of the many other nutrients eggs have. Avoiding fats is not recommended for an antiaging diet, because fats are vital to health and should be eaten in as wide a variety as you can. A better way would be to vary the oils and fats you eat and to replace high-fat foods with lower fat alternatives. Skim milk instead of whole milk, for instance, liquid vegetable oils instead of hard cooking fat, and low-fat cheeses instead of full fat.

Finally, carbohydrates should complete the balance of your diet in the form of complex carbohydrates such as wholemeal bread, pasta, or pulses. Replace foods laden with sugar with starchy and fiber-rich foods like bread, whole grains, cereals, rice, fruits, and vegetables. Most American women in their 30s do not eat enough fruits and vegetables. The slow metabolism of fiber-rich foods helps blood sugars stabilize, pushes cholesterol levels down, and keeps the colon clean. Fiber also contains many vital nutrients which are absorbed slowly into the blood stream. In contrast, when refined foods or supplements are metabolized they are released quickly and compete for absorption. That is why it is always better to obtain your nutrients from your diet rather than from supplements.

Free Radicals: The Enemy

Oxidation is essential for life. It is the process whereby molecules and proteins combine with oxygen to release energy essential for mental and physical energy. Free radicals are, unfortunately, the byproduct of this process. They are also created by the body in response to the food we eat, ultraviolet light, ozone, tobacco smoke, vehicle emissions, and pollutants. Free radicals damage molecules which then go on to injure and attack cells in the body, leaving them susceptible to potential toxins.

Many experts believe that free radical reactions underlie the deterioration that is the hallmark of aging in all individuals, however healthy. In our youth we are firing on all cylinders, but as our bodies slowly become depleted of essential nutrients in our 30s, free radicals take hold. Free radicals not only cause illnesses like cancer, senility, and strokes, they can be prematurely aging.

We are all oxidizing away like an apple that has been bitten and gradually grows brown. The damage manifests itself in aging events like wrinkles, dry skin, and so on. But we can fight free radicals with nutrients or nutrient-derived enzymes that neutralize them. It is believed that a diet rich in antioxidants can harness much of the destructive free radical energy.

Antioxidants

Our natural defenses against free radicals are antioxidants. The most important food-derived antioxidants are beta carotene (the nontoxic part of vitamin A), vitamins C and E, as well as certain B compounds, and the minerals selenium, manganese, copper, and zinc.

Nutritional experts suggest that we should increase the amount of antioxidants we eat to keep in good health. There is a big difference at present between the RDA allowance for certain vitamins which ensure that deficiency diseases, like beriberi or rickets, don't occur and the large amount now being suggested to prevent degenerative changes in the body. The amount of vitamin E, for example, needed to give antioxidant protection is seven times the standard RDA. Since many vitamins and minerals taken in large doses can be toxic (see "Warning") caution is advised.

Following are some antiaging antioxidants you might want to consider increasing in your diet or taking as a supplement.

Vitamin A is found in whole milk products, fish, liver, margarine, eggs, carrots, orange/yellow fruits, and dark-green leafy vegetables. Beta carotene, the nontoxic form of vitamin A, is a prime defense against cancer. In general, though, it is an all-around strengthener of the immune system.

Vitamin C is found in any yellow/orange or deep green fruit or vegetable, in particular carrots, spinach, tomato, sprouts, strawberries, watercress, sweet potatoes, broccoli, apricots, peaches, and pink grapefruit. It seems that to forestall the impact of aging, you can never have enough vitamin C. Vitamin C strengthens the immune system and can stop you from getting so many colds. It fights fatigue and gives energy. Some studies show that too much vitamin C can cause diarrhea and ill health, but this is debatable. If you smoke, your requirement for vitamin C rises threefold.

Vitamin E is found in vegetable oils, wheat germ, nuts, seeds, whole grains, legumes, leafy vegetables, lettuce, and egg yolks. Antioxidizing action helps keep arteries strong, boosts the immune system, relieves menstrual problems, fights aging, and protects against cancer. Too much vitamin E can lead to diarrhea and cramps, so it is best to keep within the RDA.

Selenium is found in seeds and nuts as well as seafood and whole grains. It is key in warding off infections.

Zinc is found in brewer's yeast, beans, egg yolks, and shellfish. Zinc promotes a strong immune system and helps skin look youthful. It also protects the liver and helps absorb vitamin E.

Manganese-rich foods include whole grains, dried peas and beans, and leafy green vegetables. Manganese is good for bones, fertility, and mental alertness.

Copper is found in green vegetables, milk, meat, and bread. Copper is important for the metabolism of zinc and for a feeling of well-being.

Other Antiaging Recommendations

To ensure that you maintain optimum health in the 30s, the following vitamins and minerals and extra supplements are also worth considering if you think you might be deficient.

Vitamin B_{12} is important for the digestive system and nervous system. It can therefore help with digestive problems and is supposed to help us think more clearly. It can also prevent anemia. Most multivitamins should contain vitamin B_{12} in sufficient amounts. It is found in meat, fish, and dairy products as well. Vegetarians tend to be deficient in this vitamin.

Vitamin B_6 boosts the immune system, and relieves water retention and menstrual problems. Most multivitamins contain sufficient B_6, but it is better to get it from food sources like eggs, fish, meat, beans, broccoli, potatoes, and soybeans.

B vitamins help skin, eyes, hair, liver, gut, brain, and mouth stay healthy. They are an essential part of an antiaging diet and are found in nuts, seeds, milk, eggs, leafy vegetables, cheeses, broccoli, bananas, liver, and peanuts. To work most effectively B vitamins must be taken together. They are especially important for women taking oral contraceptives.

Folic acid is important for cell production and healthy skin. It is found in leafy green vegetables, chicken, liver, and kidneys. It is essential for all pregnant women. For aging, folic acid is believed to be a brain food. The RDA is 400 mg a day.

Vitamin P aids the absorption of vitamin C. Foods rich in vitamin P include apricots, berries, and citrus fruit.

Vitamin Q is essential to the extraction of energy from nutrients. With aging and illness, deficiency in vitamin Q can cause weight retention, heart and circulation difficulties, and problems with the immune system. Foods high in vitamin Q include fatty, oily fish, nuts, and green leafy vegetables.

Calcium is needed for healthy teeth and gums and keeps the skeleton strong in later life. Good food sources include milk, cheese, yogurt, green vegetables, spinach, almonds, and sesame seeds.

Magnesium assists in the absorption of both calcium and potassium. If your diet is deficient in calcium you might show signs of nervousness and irritability. Foods rich in magnesium include figs, nuts, apples, whole-wheat grains, and seeds.

Potassium is crucial to body function. Deficiency can cause bloating, fatigue, dry skin, muscle weakness, and slow reflexes. Potassium is found in a wide variety of foods including bananas, oranges, tomatoes, mushrooms, potatoes, eggs, and oatmeal.

Acidophilus is a substance that helps us digest and absorb nutrients. It is bacteria we produce in our stomachs that has beneficial effects. Stress, illness, and drugs can all disrupt the right level of bacteria in our stomach and the natural source of acidophilus in live yogurts can be beneficial.

Carnitine helps process fat. The main food source is from animal foods, so vegetarians might be advised to take a supplement.

Glutathione is another substance that, like carnitine, is produced from amino acids. It is present in the liver, where it breaks down harmful toxins from what we eat, so a glutathione deficiency can accelerate the aging process. The body can continue to manufacture this substance provided there are no vitamin and mineral deficiencies.

It is a surprise that so many thirtysomething American women don't know about the benefits of omega acids and are in fact deficient in them. As mentioned previously, women in their 30s and 40s need a diet rich in omega 3 and omega 6 fatty acids. It seems we get enough omega 6 from food sources like rice bran and peanut, olive, coconut, soy, and flaxseed oil, but not enough omega 3, found in sea vegetables, green leafy vegetables and fresh coldwater fish like mackerel and herring.

To Supplement or Not to Supplement

Although supplements have been suggested, it is best to get your nutrients the natural way, from the food you eat. Eat a wide variety of foods in moderation. Don't think of food in terms of good or bad. Think of food as a way of keeping your body and mind functioning optimally.

Vitamin supplements are now readily available. Almost half of all Americans take them at some point in their lives. The trouble with supplements, though, is that they encourage pill popping and not a lifestyle change. In your 30s supplements should really be a last resort. With your digestive system still robust you should be able to get all the nutrients you need from a balanced diet and indeed many experts believe that this is the best way to get them. The process of digestion is still a mystery. Food is metabolized more efficiently and substances are produced that supplements cannot manufacture.

In an ideal world, you would get all the nutrients you need from the food you eat, have good digestion, never get stressed out, and never lose a night's sleep. Unfortunately we don't live in this ideal world and in some cases supplements may be advisable as a last resort. If you must take a supplement make sure that what you are taking is safe and consult your doctor or a qualified nutritionist to ensure that the dosage is correct. This is especially the case if you think you need more than the RDA for vitamins and minerals. In most cases taking a multivitamin and mineral supplement is better than individual supplements because research has shown that in order for specific vitamins and minerals to be properly metabolized all the other vitamins and minerals need to be present too.

Warning

When taking any form of supplement, always check with your doctor or a nutritional expert to make sure it is safe. Overdose of certain vitamins can be toxic.

- **Vitamin A**—Can cause brain and liver damage if taken in high doses. Dangerous if taken during pregnancy.
- **Beta carotene**—Large doses are nontoxic but they can turn the skin yellow and cause menstrual irregularity.
- **Vitamin B$_3$**—Large doses can cause hot flashes and liver problems.
- **Vitamin D**—Large doses can cause nausea, headache, diarrhea, and loss of appetite.
- **Vitamin E**—Large doses can cause nausea, headache, fainting, and heart palpitations.
- **Calcium**—Large doses can cause constipation and interfere with the absorption of other minerals.
- **Selenium**—Large doses can nausea, diarrhea, and nerve damage.
- **Zinc**—Large doses can cause nausea and vomiting.
- **Iron**—Large doses can increase the risk of heart disease.

Herbal Supplements

Natural or herbal supplements that claim to delay the aging process or relieve symptoms of aging are gaining in popularity. As with vitamin and mineral supplements, use them with caution and seek expert advice before you begin a course of treatment. Following are a few of the most popular supplements currently available.

- *Bee propolis* can stimulate the immune system and is good for a number of common ailments. It is made from the substances bees use to construct their hives.
- *Burdock root* and *red clover* cleanse the bloodstream.

- A cup of *chamomile tea* daily is a great digestive aid with considerable therapeutic effects.
- *Dong quai* is an herb that is supposed to be good for hot flashes and vaginal dryness.
- *Echinacea* is an herb that can stimulate the production of white cells and is good to use if you are feeling run down.
- *Evening primrose oil.* Many women in perimenopause find relief from evening primrose oil. It can help balance fluctuating hormone levels.
- *Green tea* is a powerful antioxidant recommended for anyone concerned about premature aging.
- *Ginseng and ginkgo* extracts give energy, improve brain function, and increase circulation. (Do not take ginkgo if you have high blood pressure.)
- *Horsetail,* taken in tea or extract form, provides bone-strengthening silicon.
- *Milk thistle* promotes healthy liver function.
- *Nettle* is full of vital vitamins.
- *St. John's wort* is used for almost every ailment that is stress- or depression-related. It can interfere with the absorption of other minerals, so use with care.
- *Tea tree oil* is used to treat skin conditions and for soothing vaginal infections when added to a bath.
- *Wild yam* contains natural steroids which have a rejuvenating effect.
- Production of *melatonin* tapers off as we get older. The hormone may alleviate symptoms of perimenopause. Melatonin is found in small amounts in rice, barley and corn. It is also available in drug stores in pill, capsule, and liquid form. (There are no long term studies on melatonin supplements, so use with caution.)
- *DHEA.* As we age, levels of DHEA hormone decline. It is only to be taken as a supplement under professional advice.

Water

Don't forget the most important nutrient of all that your body needs—water. "Water is considered the universal solvent. It is vital to all stages of life, and of course perimenopause is no exception" (Gittleman, p. 167).

Our bodies are about two-thirds water, so the intake and distribution of fluid is vital. If the body is deprived of water, blood volume is reduced and blood does not circulate to the tissues as effectively. This leads to fatigue and maybe even dizziness. You won't look fresh and energetic and your skin will certainly look dry. Water helps lubricate dehydrated and parched tissues as well as aiding the body in eliminating waste. It keeps skin glowing and your cells and systems working and it delivers vitamins, minerals, and other nutrients to all your organs. For glands to secrete hormones and for the liver to break down and excrete toxins you need to be hydrated. Drinking plenty of water will also help fluid retention because it will be forcing water through your system more efficiently.

Women need to ensure that they drink enough water. Six to eight glasses a day is recommended. It would be a good idea to have a bottle of water with you at all times. Drink a glass of water before you eat a meal to make sure that your hunger pangs are not dehydration. Always have water with you when you exercise or fly, and drink pure water rather than carbonated water, tea, coffee, sodas, and other sugary drinks because these can actually dehydrate you more.

If you find drinking all that water difficult, try adding flavoring to your water. Lemon or grapefruit juice can be refreshing.

It can be hard in this modern age of preservatives and additives to know exactly if the water you get from your tap or bottle is pure. Distilling water removes trace minerals, some of which your body needs. You might consider purifying water in the home with a Doulton ceramic water filter, which can be ordered from Uni-Key at 800-888-4353.

Alcohol

Drinking in excess in your 30s can take about 15 years off your life expectancy. A woman who drinks excessively over long periods of time will, if the addiction is not checked, look older than her non-drinking contemporaries. Her skin is likely to look pale and as alcohol is dehydrating, it will look dry and wrinkly too. She will appear weak or even have a nervous shake. Her face will be swollen and her eyes bloodshot and she will have a bloated stomach because alcohol damages the liver.

Light drinking on the other hand may actually improve some aspects of your health. This is a conflicting and difficult message to get across to our generation, who know all about the dangers of drinking: murderous drunk driving, liver disease, and addiction. Most doctors prefer us not to know that a few drinks can be beneficial, fearful that the subtleties of the message will be missed and it will just give excessive drinkers another chance to indulge.

The problem is that it is so hard to define what light drinking is. So far research is showing that enjoying one or two drinks a day won't harm your health and may even benefit it. The harm starts after those two drinks and escalates dramatically.

At one or two drinks blood pressure stays low, liver damage is unlikely, and there is a direct protective effect on the heart and circulatory system, with no ill effects on the brain. Larger amounts of alcohol, however, can raise blood pressure, potentially damage the liver and heart, cause digestive and fertility problems, and affect mental function. There is also a link between excessive drinking and breast cancer. Women in their 30s who are social drinkers may be drinking far more than they think and are totally unaware that there is a big difference between the sexes and how much they can safely consume. Women can only drink about half as much as men before risking their health. If you already have one or two drinks a day this won't do any harm, but you need to be aware that any more puts you in the danger zone.

Individuals who should be careful about how much they drink are pregnant and nursing moms (alcohol can stunt a child's development), those with a history of alcohol problems, and those who may have inherited a tendency to alcoholism. For the rest of us a small amount of alcohol may make us feel and look better, but too much can be deadly. Once again, moderation is the key.

Unfortunately, statistics show that the number of women drinking and smoking is on the increase. Women in their 30s, especially those who work, are not taking care of themselves and drinking far too much. Not only will the addiction age them visibly, but even more worrying is the damage being done inside the body. The long-term risks to health are considerable. Excessive drinking will cause metabolic change and weaken the immune system. The lining of the stomach will be destroyed. Infertility and loss of libido are likely. Blood pressure will be elevated and the heart will get progressively weaker. The liver can get so damaged it can't absorb nutrients anymore. Alcohol prevents the absorption of fat, so the liver will get clogged with fat. There is also a high risk of diabetes.

Alcohol damages your system. Good nutrition can help reverse some of this damage, but if you keep drinking to excess liver damage will be irreversible. Making sure you get an adequate intake of vitamins, especially the B vitamins, amino acids, vitamin C, calcium, magnesium, and zinc, which all strengthen the liver, will help.

If you begin to depend on your drink on a daily basis and find it hard to stop after a few drinks, you may have a drinking problem. The safe limit for women is fourteen units a week, but each of us has an individual response to alcohol. (One unit of alcohol is a 3-oz. glass of wine or ½ pint of beer.) Bear in mind, though, that before the outward signs of alcohol manifest themselves the alcohol is already in your blood stream. If you are addicted nothing short of total abstinence may work, but if you like to have a drink the sensible thing is to make sure you eat before you drink; to eat a healthy, nutritious diet; to drink lots of water; to avoid drinking if you are on medication; and to restrict the number of days that you drink so that your system gets time to recover.

Nicotine

There is absolutely no doubt about it. If you smoke in your 30s you are going to look years older than your nonsmoking contemporaries.

Your bones will be weaker, you will have more lines on your face, and you will probably enter menopause a few years earlier. Smoking can decrease blood supply to the skin, cutting off the normal supply of oxygen. It also makes the skin look less supple and gives it a yellowish, leathery tinge. Just as with alcohol, women need fewer cigarettes to get comparable levels of nicotine in their blood and they don't metabolize it as quickly as men. Smoking increases your risk of cancer, heart disease, and lung, throat, respiratory passage, and esophagus disease. It also affects the reproductive organs and increases risk of cancer of the cervix. Women who smoke when they are pregnant run higher risks of miscarriage and stillbirth. Smoking has also been linked to incontinence caused by repeated coughing weakening the pelvic floor. Smoking is especially dangerous if you are on the contraceptive pill because both smoking and the contraceptive pill deplete the body's essential nutrients.

Not only that, but you are more likely to have an early menopause, to contract lung cancer, or to have a heart attack than nonsmokers. Smoking will also give you wrinkles, yellowish, gray-looking skin, bloodshot eyes, yellow teeth, and breath like a dirty ashtray. So why do so many of us in our 30s do it?

Simple. We think it will keep us slim. Instead of a chocolate bar we have a cigarette. We have all read somewhere that smoking speeds up metabolism. It's debatable whether smoking does actually keep the weight off, but what is the point of losing a few pounds if you get wrinkles, bad breath, a hacking cough, and lack energy?

Any woman who is concerned about aging in her 30s would be advised to give up smoking. This won't be easy if you have become addicted and are worrying about your weight. Smoking does raise metabolic rate and instead of snacking many women smoke. Withdrawal can also create carbohydrate cravings. But with a carefully thought-out diet plan and lots of exercise, it won't take long for your metabolism to adjust.

You can give up smoking if you really want the best for yourself. There are many ways to stop smoking. You may decide to use nicotine replacement or join a group or go for acupuncture. The cold turkey approach, however, is often the most effective. It only takes a few days for the nicotine to leave your system and any cravings after that are due to habit.

Whatever method you decide always remember when the going gets tough that you are undoing all the damage that smoking has done to your body and that giving up smoking will make you look and feel years younger.

There are so many reasons to give up smoking, but the most important one is that you deserve better. You deserve to feel better. You deserve to sleep, eat, and look better. You deserve to age better.

Substance Abuse

Those of us who experimented with drugs in our 20s should know by now that drugs, like heroin for example, can be prematurely aging and have life-threatening side effects. We may not know, however, that some of the other so-called lighter drugs can also have terrible risks. Ecstasy can cause brain damage. Cocaine can destroy your nose.

Any drug that becomes addictive, painkillers or sleeping pills for example, can age you by destroying the delicate balance of the body. All drugs are dangerous. The only one which seems to have any kind of positive effect, if taken with moderation and care, is marijuana or cannabis. Doctors have used it to ease pain and to relax patents.

Caffeine

The caffeine in coffee, tea, chocolate, and cola gives many of us a kick-start because it is a mild stimulant. It may have good short-term effects, but the long term effects of irritability, insomnia, and mood swings are not so pleasant.

Caffeine is addictive, as most of us in our 30s know. Now and again is fine but if you find yourself drinking several cups of strong coffee a day you are putting your system under stress that is aging. Caffeine is a diuretic. It can make us get dehydrated, it blocks the absorption of water soluble tissues in the body, overworks the kidneys, and makes us age faster, but despite all that many of us just can't give up our daily Starbucks (or two or three).

Like most addictions the more caffeine you have the more you need to feel the stimulant effect. With nutrients depleted and tissues dehydrated you are slowly damaging your body. Decaffeinated drinks can sometimes be as bad as caffeinated ones. There are lots of caffeine-free drinks available now and if it is really unrealistic for you to give up your coffee, drink it in moderation and drink lots of water to keep hydrated.

Junk Food

Junk food, in my opinion, is any kind of food that lacks the necessary nutrients to keep us healthy. It is never fresh. It often contains a lot of sugar, fat, salt, artificial flavoring, and chemicals—chocolate and potato chips, for example. Fast food or anything that is fried or that comes in a packet with all the nutrients dried out of it is junk food. Sugary drinks are junk food, too.

People who live on a diet of junk food are often overweight but malnourished, because the food they eat does not give their bodies the essential nutrients they need. They won't look healthy, either, and the chances are that their hair, skin, and nails look lackluster.

It may have been "all right" in your 20s to live on chocolate bars and hamburgers but in your 30s your body won't let you get away with it anymore. A diet that is deficient in vitamins and minerals will eventually damage your heath. It can make you vulnerable to the attack of aging free radicals, cause indigestion, raise cholesterol, raise blood pressure, clog your arteries, and increase the risk of diabetes and obesity.

Over half of the ten leading causes of death in America are diet related. You can quite literally eat yourself to a state of ill health. Cancer, heart attacks, and other causes of ill health associated with old age are diet related. When the role of food in degenerative illness was discovered 30 years ago, the focus was on what we shouldn't be eating. Cholesterol, alcohol, caffeine, and red meat were all put under the spotlight. Today, however, the focus has shifted to how our health can be impacted by what we should be eating.

Eating a healthy balanced diet in the 30s and avoiding junk food is crucial if you want to improve your health and vitality and delay the aging process. You don't have to spend hours planning and preparing your meals or spend lots of money on supplements or never eat another chocolate bar again, you just need to eat a wide variety of foods in moderation and make sure you include plenty of the right types of food that can help you look your best. And in the process you will discover an antiaging strategy that actually works.

Chapter 9
An Antiaging Lifestyle

There is no magic elixir of youth, but eating a healthy, balanced diet in your 30s will help delay the aging process. In combination with a balanced diet, though, regular exercise and stress management are also beneficial if you want to feel and look energetic and vital.

Inactivity

Inactivity in your 30s will age you fast. If you spent your 20s running around for your job in junior positions, being promoted to more senior positions in the 30s can mean a more sedentary lifestyle. At first this may come as a pleasant relief, but unless you ensure that you keep active in your spare time your health could suffer.

Lack of exercise will make you feel less energetic and vital. If you haven't got zest you will seem far older than you are. Zest and vitality are the most youthful characteristics any woman can have. They transcend age barriers. A woman without zest seems old even if she is in her 20s. A woman with zest and vitality is like a breath of fresh air. There is an energy about everything she does. A youthful energy that makes her attractive, charismatic, and ageless.

Most of us exercise to look more toned or to lose weight, but the antiaging benefits of exercise are far more important than an improvement in how you look. One of the most effective ways to improve your health is by exercising regularly. It should be a top health priority at any age.

In our 30s we start to lose strength and power at the rate of 1 to 2 percent a year. Exercise can help delay that process and actually increase the strength of our muscles. Exercise encourages body awareness and weight loss. It decreases muscular tension and joint pain, can prevent osteoporosis, increase circulation, improve lung capacity, enhance bowel movement, help control and prevent incontinence, lessen lower back pain, prevent swollen ankles, generate warmth, heighten alertness, help with insomnia, alleviate depression, improve cholesterol profile, decrease the risk of diabetes, heart disease and breast and colon cancer, ease the discomforts of PMS, regulate blood sugar, fight colds and infections, and help build bones and calorie-burning muscles, thus promoting weight loss. It makes us feel more energetic, removes toxic substances from the body, and improves posture and body image. It can help reduce stress, anxiety, and depression because it releases endorphins, which can improve your mood. It can lower the level of pulse-quickening hormones released during stress and can stimulate a feeling of well-being. Even a 30-minute walk around the block can reduce anxiety.

And if all that weren't enough, exercise can also make a woman feel sexier and live longer. It "improves strength, sleeping patterns, and self-esteem," says Donna Meltzer, M.D., a clinical assistant professor in the department of family medicine at State University of New York (*Fit Pregnancy*, Spring 1999, p. 103.)

Fit for Life

We all age differently. Some of us keep our bodies in shape but our faces get lined. Others have young-looking faces but flabby bodies. Some worry more about external appearance but neglect feeling strong and vibrant from the inside. Others think that keeping slim is more important than keeping fit.

Genetics and good luck do play a part, but your attitude to your body plays a huge part too. In our 30s if we want to look and feel healthy we really have to stop fretting about our weight or our size and concentrate on our fitness levels. Keeping slim does not equal looking young or looking fit. Women who stay unnaturally thin age badly and more noticeably without the extra flesh to give skin its elasticity. Bear in mind, though, too much flab can be aging. If you can pinch more than an inch or two on your waist then you have flab to lose.

Being fit and toned with a great posture and an energetic pace is far more important than being thin or just looking good on the outside. Women who are fit and who lead an active lifestyle have a beauty that is timeless and a vitality that is infectious.

An Exercise Plan

Most of us in our 30s will have grown up hearing about the benefits of exercise. Fitness gurus and personalities literally clutter the media. We may even have been lucky enough to see our parents jumping on the bandwagon, ensuring that exercise is a part of our lives. If you already exercise regularly and enjoy it you don't need to be told how important exercise is and how beneficial it is for your mind, body, and spirit. Exercise is a part of your life, like brushing your teeth or combing your hair. If you are in your 30s and not exercising regularly you need to understand that exercise is the best thing you can do for yourself. It will improve body image and build self-esteem. For weight loss, increased energy, physical strength and an overall feeling of well-being, exercise is an antiaging must.

If you haven't got the time or the inclination to join a gym you can design your own exercise program. Your program should include aerobic activity, strength training, and stretching.

Lack of aerobic exercise is the main cause of weight gain and circulatory problems. Aerobic exercise means exercising regularly with oxygen repeatedly for an extend period of time so that your body starts burning fat and blood pumps faster around your body. You should be out of breath but not so much that you can't carry on a conversation while you exercise. If you exercise too hard you won't be exercising aerobically. Aerobic exercises include brisk walking, jogging, swimming, cycling, rowing, stair climbing, aerobic dance classes, step classes, and boxing. Aerobic exercise for around 45 minutes three to five times a week should be enough. If you stop after just 20 minutes you are unlikely to get most of the aerobic benefits of sustained exercise, which encourages fat burning.

In addition to aerobic exercise, strength training is important too. As well as helping you maintain your weight strength training helps fight the effects of aging, since we lose muscle strength as we age. Strength training also gives your body shape and tone and will give you more energy. Training for strength means working your muscles harder than you normally do with lifting, pulling, and pushing. Most gyms would be able to help you with a strength training program with weights or machines, but there are many alternatives that achieve the same results. Yoga, pilates, or calisthenics are examples. Or you might like to do simple strengthening exercises yourself, such as squats, lunges, press-ups, and sit-ups.

Strengthening exercises should be done for about 30 minutes three times a week with rest days in between for the muscles to recuperate.

If you are like most women in their 30s and you want to have a long, lean, fit body, stretching and lengthening your body is vital. Calf stretching, when you feel the stretch in your calf by leaning against a wall or pressing your heels down on a step, is important to do before aerobic exercise. Lying on your back and drawing your knees into your chest will stretch the lower back. There are also stretches for the front and back of your thighs, your chest, hips, shoulders, and arms. One of the easiest and most beneficial stretches is the whole body stretch. Put your hands up in the air, rise on your toes, and stretch as hard as you can, as if you were trying to reach something. Stretching is an activity you can do daily.

But what about those of us who really don't like exercise or simply have not got the time? The answer is to find an exercise you enjoy. If you dread your workouts, stop them and do something different. Perhaps you might feel more committed to exercise if you found an activity that was social and included other people, like dancing or exercise classes. If you hate gyms try to incorporate toning and strengthening exercises into your daily life. For example, you can tighten your buttocks at different times during the day or try to improve your posture. Make your daily life a little more active and don't sit around too much. Putting more energy into everyday chores like housework or gardening can burn calories and build muscle tone too.

Many women who hate exercise actually find that they enjoy walking. Walking really doesn't seem like exercise, but the benefits of a regular walking program are incredible. You can walk indoors or outdoors. Try to start including it into your daily schedule and if possible it might even become your means of transport. Make sure you don't have heavy bags when you walk and that you wear supportive walking shoes. Aim to try to walk at a pace that makes your heart beat a little faster; if fat burning is your aim, try to walk at least five times a week. You can walk every day, as long as you don't push yourself. The question of how often you can walk is less important than how long you walk for. If your schedule is too tight for long walks there are still benefits to several short walks a day. Even a few minutes of exercise a day is beneficial. Always warm up before you do any sort of exercise, however short. And remember that muscles need stretching after strengthening.

With any exercise routine, no matter how much you are committed, expect to feel bored with it from time to time. If this is the case try to vary your schedule and add lots of variety. Mix your workouts and try something new. Too many rest days will make you lose condition but do make sure that you have regular rest days for your body to recover.

The important thing is to listen to your body. Many of us in our 30s are overworked or stressed and have made ignoring the warning signals our bodies give us a habit. If you feel any pain, tiredness, dizziness, headaches, blurred vision, breathlessness, or an uneven heartbeat, stop. Your body is speaking to you all the time. Listen to it. It is far wiser than you are.

Posture

As we get older our posture changes. Years of sitting and standing incorrectly and wearing high heels have their effect. Postural quirks become more noticeable as the spine adapts to the demands of our lifestyle.

If we want to look and feel fit in our 30s it is time to pay attention to our posture. We can't get away with slumping shoulders and stooping anymore. "Good posture carries off clothes to the best effort, lends ease and freedom to movement, and counteracts the dejected downward slant of the shoulders that is in every way aging. It is what, quite literally, enables us to grow older gracefully. It is the link between fitness and fashion, the point at which the aesthetics of health and those of beauty meet" (Hutton, p. 195).

In our 30s improving our posture will have great health benefits. Good posture is critical to our well-being. It makes us look taller, thinner, and more sure of ourselves. Perhaps from childhood you have been told to hold your back straight and head high if for no other reason than to look self-assured. However, as an adult physical comfort actually becomes contingent on your posture. Too much slumping as we walk, sit, or eat will potentially put undue pressure on the spine and aging back trouble and joint pain are virtually inevitable.

But What Is Good Posture?

Good posture has nothing to do with the old school rigidity of pulling in your stomach and puffing your chest out. Good posture is about looking effortlessly pulled up. It is about ease of movement and freedom and using the minimum amount of effort to keep the body upright. Life can be stressful and it can be hard to obtain this ideal. We are needlessly tensing and straining our bodies all day long, which wastes energy. We don't observe proper body mechanics and pull the whole out of line. Small wonder that we get "unexplained" aches and pains, sleepless nights, and mood swings. All too often improper body mechanics are causing the tension.

When we start to become aware of the degree of tension in our bodies can we begin to make positive changes. Once we stop all the distortions we may well find that aches and pains disappear, that we are all a little taller, have more energy, and feel better.

When muscles relax we return energy to our bodies, according to Oriental traditions of medicine who call this energy Qi. Qi travels through the body along pathways, and when Qi gets blocked ill health occurs. Energy and well-being can be restored by getting the energy flowing again by releasing the tension we store away in our muscles.

Proprioception is the term used for the process that keeps the body in a state of alignment. Muscle spindles alongside the muscle fibers supply the brain with a continual flow of information via the spinal cord and nerves and in turn receive the instructions to keep us in balance. There are various techniques which can help us tune into this inner balance. Yoga, tai chi, martial arts, and Alexander technique are examples.

Realignment methods may have different philosophies behind them but the goal is often the same: a free, supple, lengthened body that resists the tendency we have to contract, which causes many of the discomforts we wrongly associate with getting older. Common to all these methods is the emphasis on doing the minimum so that only the relevant muscles are brought into play. As physical effort diminishes, mental clarity and inner harmony increase. We understand our bodies from the inside out rather than the outside in. We begin to appreciate just how remarkable our body is and are less self-critical as we concentrate on whole body awareness.

If you don't want to take up a realignment method to improve your posture, there are ways you can work on your posture yourself. First of all you need to become aware that the muscles of alignment are situated at the back of our body not the front. That is why sucking in our tummies or pulling back our shoulders often doesn't improve our shape. The muscles at the front of the body are not meant to be stabilizing but the muscles that run along the back and spine and legs are. As we are not used to using these muscles, at first they may need retraining. This may explain why you may find it hard to stand balanced on both feet rather than shifting from one to the other, or to sit with legs uncrossed rather than with legs crossed.

Fortunately, once you start thinking of the back to front way, muscles don't take long to get back into operation and it won't seem so tiring. Once you get used to lengthening, the stomach naturally flattens and your shape improves.

To do a quick check on your posture have a look at yourself sideways in a mirror. Try to tuck your bottom under and pull upward. Lift your head and chin up and feel as if someone is pulling you from the center of your head with a string. If you compare how you look now you will realize how slumped you normally are. You'll also see how good posture can take pounds off you and makes you look more confident and poised.

Alongside posture, proper body mechanics is also important to avoid strain and tension. When bending or lifting, plant the feet firmly apart and bend the knees so that the back stays long. Hold an object you are lifting close to you and lift it by straightening your knees, not your back. Pull up when you sit, and try to avoid crossing your legs. This can be a hard habit to break but if continued it will really weaken the lower back muscles. Work at desks that are the right height for you and that help you keep your back long. When driving make sure knees are slightly higher than your hips. And if you must wear high heels wear them for short periods only. High heels shift the center of gravity forward and distort your posture and put the body under tremendous strain.

Eastern Disciplines

Eastern disciplines like yoga and tai chi are becoming increasingly popular in the west. One of the great advantages is that they can be continued well into old age. Yoga classes still tend to be more popular with the older age group, but interest among thirtysomethings is growing.

Yoga is the ideal antiaging exercise. It works against gravity and always stretches and lengthens the body and never jars or shortens joints. It keeps the body supple, improves circulation and strength, and does wonders for your posture. Yoga exercise should never be forced and should be done slowly and gently with deep breathing. Strength comes from the time spent holding poses. If you want to start a yoga routine make sure you join a class with an experienced instructor.

Stress Management

Maturity brings with it added responsibilities. Never before has there been so much pressure on us as far as work and family are concerned. We are expected to know what we want, to be in a settled relationship, to have bought that house. If we haven't "settled" we need to decide what our priorities are. If we have settled we need to decide if this is the life we want or if changes should be made. On top of all this parents may need extra care, work may be more pressurized, finances may be tight, and friends and partners more demanding. Without realizing it, our busy lives could be a major source of stress.

Stress puts the body and mind in a state of crisis. It is aging.

Stress occurs when there is an imbalance between the demands of your life and your ability to cope with these demands. Continued stress over a long period of time will affect all your body systems. To cope with stress the body will secrete stress hormones into the blood stream. When stress is prolonged too much stress hormone is released and this will affect all the body systems. It will exhaust the adrenal glands, upset the balance of hormones, deplete the body's resources and produce fatigue, changes in appetite, insomnia, depression and deprive the brain of oxygen, killing off brain cells. It can diminish the body's immune system, making you more vulnerable to disease. It may also bring on hypertension, a recognized factor in heart disease, and some cancers.

Stress can be caused by major life changes, such as divorce or the death of a loved one, but even a busy life or changes in routine, eating habits, travel arrangements, or place of residence will challenge the body as it tries to adapt to the new way of doing things. Sometimes even activities considered pleasurable, such as weddings or holidays, can be stressful. Infection, fever, exposure to hot and cold, increased physical activity, certain drugs or addictions to smoking, alcohol, or drugs will also cause the body stress.

Our thoughts, feelings, and moods can be stressful. Emotional stress as well as physical stress can affect the secretion of stress hormones into the bloodstream which in turn affects sex hormones and blood sugar levels. Hormonal imbalance will accelerate the age process. We need a certain amount of challenge and stress in our life, but it should be a positive kind of stress that does not make us feel uncomfortable. It is negative stress, stress that is exhausting and draining, that results in anxiety and eventual mental and physical breakdown. This is the kind of stress to avoid. If we cannot avoid it we need to learn to deal with it in a positive way.

We all react to stress in different ways. Stress levels tend to be highest among those of us who feel that our lives are out of our control. In the words of Joan Borysenko in *Minding the Body, Mending the Mind*, it all depends on our constitutions. "Most of us will feel that life is out of control in some way. Whether we see this as a temporary situation, whose resolution will add to our store of knowledge and experience, or as one more threat demonstrating life's dangers, is the most crucial question both for the quality of our life and our physical health" (1987, p. 16).

Stress reduction plays an important part in delaying the aging process. If stress levels are high, stress reduction must be one of the first priorities. You don't need to take a long vacation or change your life dramatically. Eating a healthy balanced diet or exercising regularly may be all that is needed. Looking older than you are can be stress related. Stress levels tend to be high in the 30s as we take on more commitments at work and at home. Stress reduction should be a priority.

The subject of stress management could fill a book. In brief, eating a balanced healthy diet, exercising regularly, getting enough sleep, learning to relax, relating to others, helping others, finding your sense of humor, and cultivating a positive outlook will all help you reduce the amount of stress in your life and look years younger.

Rest

Getting the right amount of rest will reduce the amount of stress in your life and keep your youthful looks. Eating late, drinking alcohol, smoking, exercising before bed, and going to bed after midnight can rob you of restful sleep. Stress and anxiety are also sleep robbers.

Lack of sleep and too much sleep will make you feel fatigued and stressed. Sleep is biologically necessary. Most of us need around eight hours a night, and if we don't get it in our 30s we will not function well and it will affect our mood. Too much sleep will also get you out of condition so you need to discover what is best for you. Sleep is vital for optimum brainpower; without it we would quickly become depressed, irritated, stressed, and fuzzy-headed. Restful sleep is vital because of its rejuvenating qualities. It encourages the production of certain hormones that keep you looking youthful.

We do need less sleep as we age. About eight hours is right in our 30s, but each one of us will be different. Some may need less, some may need more. Chronic fatigue, if you can't deal with it through stress reduction and exercise, may need medical attention. Feeling tired all the time in your 30s is not a natural state to be in. There could be autoimmune problems or mood disorders, such as depression. So if fatigue is becoming a way of life make sure you consult a doctor.

Insomnia, the inability to fall asleep, does seem to get more common as we get older. If this is the case you need to identify the stresses in your life which are keeping you awake. If you can deal with them, restful sleep may follow. If you can't deal with them or your sleep problems persist, see a doctor.

Lack of sleep and too much stress can also lead to headaches. There are many sorts of headaches—from those that give you a vague sense of discomfort to those that make you wrinkle up your face in agony. Migraines are a different type of headache and are caused by a spasm of the blood vessels supplying the brain. They can be treated with some success by drugs. The occasional headache, especially after a rough night, is normal, but any headache that is persistent should be checked out immediately with a doctor. Try to note what time of day your headache occurs and what foods or activities trigger it. It could well be due to poor light, poor diet, a sedentary lifestyle, or poor vision, but it could also be the early warning signs of a stroke or brain tumor, so don't accept regular headaches as part of getting older. Consult your doctor.

Although there is no prescription that guarantees sweet sleep, lowering stress and learning how to relax will help. Sleeping, however, is not the only way to relax and find refreshment. Taking time out and doing something you enjoy is just as important as a good night's sleep. Try to concentrate more on being a human being rather than a human doing.

Relaxation

Many of us in our 30s feel that our lives are one long juggling act between work, home, and personal life. There is never enough time for anything. We certainly don't have time to relax. Hopefully, we will have better skill at time management and use the energy that we do have far more productively. But many of us still find it stressful to keep all the balls in the air at once, and compromises and decisions about how we want to live our lives have to be made.

If you do find yourself tired all the time the main reason could be lack of sleep. You could also be doing too much and relaxing too little. An overcrowded, excessive lifestyle when there is too much of everything can be aging. Moderation is key in the 30s if you want to lay the foundation stone for good health. This is not to say you shouldn't indulge now and again. We all need to let go sometimes. But too much of anything is never good. Too much food. Too much drink. Too many parties. It can also apply to things which you might think are good for you like diet and exercise. You *can* have too much of a good thing. Taking exercise programs to extremes, for example, can cause fatigue and injuries, and taking dieting too far can result in health problems too. Even too much rest can be debilitating. We need some kind of routine in our lives.

Many of us lead frantic, busy lives and when we do finally get the time to relax we don't know how. We work hard, eat fast, play competitively, and toss and turn in our sleep. Relaxation is time for you. Each of us must find different ways to relax. Walking in the fresh air, for instance, watching a movie, reading a book, seeing friends, drawing a picture, and playing an instrument are all ways to relax. Relaxation is a time when you recharge the batteries and focus on what makes you feel good. Unfortunately, so many of us tend to neglect setting aside time and space for ourselves that we have forgotten how to relax.

If you have problems relaxing you need to learn how to take time out. One way to do this is to relax your whole body slowly, muscle by muscle. There are many tapes on the market that can help you through this process. Slowing down your breathing also gives you a chance to calm down.

Techniques like meditation and yoga can also have astonishing results on women who are stressed and tense. Try this simple routine: Choose a focus word or phrase—for example, "peace" or "happy." Sit quietly and relax your body by tensing and then relaxing your muscles and breathing deeply. Say the focus word every time you exhale. If you lose concentration, simply return your thoughts to the word. Try this for just five minutes at first and then gradually increase the amount of time. Do the routine at least once a day.

Imagery, a relaxation technique similar to daydreaming, involves allowing images to drift through your mind. Try to relax and let images come to you. Listen to tapes that involve relaxation without the sounds of nature or something describing the process of relaxation.

Such relaxation exercises done regularly can slow your breathing rate, calm your brain wave rhythms, and lower your blood pressure. Yoga can also relax tense muscles, teach you better breathing, lower your blood pressure, decrease your heart rate, and divert your mind from stress.

When you feel stressed you should try counting to ten before you react or repeat some positive affirmation, such as "I am in control." Taking things a little more slowly may also help beat stress. Soothing music can be beneficial, as can soaking in a hot tub, laughing more, interacting with others, cultivating outside interests, and diversions from your usual routine. There are so many delightful ways to relax.

In our 30s many of us think of relaxation as something only older people do, as time we can't afford to lose. Rather than thinking of it as time lost, think of it as time gained that can energize you. When you return to your routine you will feel refreshed, energized, in control, and have a better perspective on things.

Relating to Others

With the disintegration of the community and family unit, loneliness, isolation, and lack of intimacy are widespread causes of stress. Partnership with people of both sexes, both sexual and nonsexual, is important for good health and stress reduction. Our lives find meaning not only through how we feel about ourselves but in our relationships with others. All living things need relationships with those of their own kind in order to be contented. No woman is an island. We need others to be happy, and we need many kinds of different relationships to feel fulfilled.

Researchers speculate that social ties might help us cope with stresses that lower our immunity. Immune cells have receptors that bind to stress hormones and when this occurs the immune cells don't work as well and we are likely to get ill.

A good way to reduce stress is by trying to build positive relationships with others. These relationships must not be ones that drain you but ones that make you feel good about yourself. In your 30s you should have a strong enough sense of self not to spend time with people who are only interested in themselves, or take you for granted. They are not friends. Also, if you believe that friendship is all about your needs being fulfilled, you are not a friend. Friendship is about giving and receiving, and is based on the capacity to accept as well as to give love and respect. A good relationship with another person should add to your sense of zest and self-worth. If people sap your energy you are mixing with the wrong kind of people.

All too often the person who is supposed to be the source of your love and inspiration and joy is the one who causes you the most stress. Those who stay youthful often seem to be successful in dealing with partners who no longer enhance their lives and finding one that does. This not only applies to partners but to friendships and work colleagues as well. Being in bad relationships of any kind causes unhappiness and vulnerability. Dr. Dean Ornish has shown in his books that happiness can strengthen the immune system and that unhappy people are likely to suffer poor health and age faster.

Women who are happy in their relationships with others tend to be less stressed and to age better. On the other hand some of us just naturally prefer solitude and find being around people stressful. If this is the case then it is better to stay solitary. You have to figure out what makes you feel good. Just remember that we develop as human beings through our emotional connections with others and we continue to need relationships with others throughout our lives.

Enjoying Life

One of the best ways to reduce stress is simply to try and have more fun with your life. If you are in a stressful situation try to think of something light and amusing. You can deal with distress by using humor; laughter really works wonders. The positive emotions associated with laughter decrease stress hormones and increase the number of immune cells. Enjoying life is so important to decreasing the effects of aging that we've devoted a whole chapter to it. Find the activities that give you pleasure and satisfaction and make enjoying life your daily practice.

Stress reduction in combination with a healthy diet and an exercise routine are the basics of a healthy lifestyle in your 30s. You may think that the 30s are too young to get serious about your health and to worry about how you will age, but they are not. Now is the ideal time to make a commitment to a lifestyle that can make you look, feel, and age better in the years to come. It just makes sense to keep your body and mind in a state of good health when signs of getting older are still subtle. In the words of fitness guru Kenneth Cooper, "It is far cheaper and more effective to maintain good health than to regain it once it is lost."

Chapter 10
Weight Management

Effective weight management should be a natural result of eating better, exercising more, and reducing stress. Unfortunately for many of us in our 30s, how much we weigh is a major cause of concern. Not being able to fit into the dress we wore to the prom makes us feel old.

In *Bridget Jones's Diary* we see the anxious thirtysomething heroine constantly obsessing about her weight. At 119 pounds she declares herself "officially thin," at 130 pounds she feels bloated and out of shape. Each day in her diary she takes note of her weight loss and weight gain, delighted when she is on a downward spiral and distressed when the weight is piling on. For Bridget anything over 120 pounds is not ideal, but despite her efforts to keep under 120 pounds, her weight fluctuates and at the end of the year she is just one pound lighter than when it started. It is clear to the reader, but apparently not to Bridget, that her body settles naturally at around 130 pounds.

Women and food. What a complicated love-hate relationship we have with it. It is the comforter, the nurturer, a way of giving and receiving affection, and if you believe the saying "you are what you eat"—a way of living. If it is so many things, why is it also something that causes fear, guilt, resentment, and shame? Why do we have this complex relationship with food? Why is dieting such torture? Because our need for food is often not physical but emotional hunger. Instead of being angry we eat, instead of feeling sad we eat, instead of feeling lonely we eat. We comfort ourselves with food. We use food to avoid addressing unresolved emotional issues. Until we can deal with these emotional issues we will continue to have problems with food.

In our quest for self many of us stumble when it comes to food. Overcoming our obsession with food and coming to terms with our body weight is a major rite of passage for women in their 30s. Only when we can say we are in control of our eating and have a balanced, healthy body image can we satisfy the real hunger for a fulfilling relationship with ourselves, others, and society. If we can't do this no amount of dieting is going to make us feel good about ourselves.

How Much Should I Weigh Now?

Like Bridget, we all have ideas about what we should or should not weigh. There really is no one answer to how much or how little every woman in her 30s should weigh or how much she should eat. We are all individuals and what one person can survive on, another cannot. What makes one woman lose weight may not make another woman lose weight. Some of us are intolerant to certain kinds of food like dairy products, sugar, and wheat, while others are not.

Your metabolic rate (the rate at which you burn food) and your body shape are determining factors when it comes to what diet suits you best for weight management. According to some experts different body shapes have different metabolisms. This is debatable, but it is certainly true that weight gained around the waist rather than the hips is more of a health risk. It is, in fact, according to some researchers an indicator of longevity and quality of life. More than 33 inches is considered a danger point for women.

Every woman's metabolism is unique to her. That is why it is so futile to compare the weight gain and loss of two women in their 30s. One may be able to eat all she wants and not put on weight while the other has to be more careful. If metabolism is efficient, food will burn quickly. If metabolism is slow, weight will pile on more quickly.

By our 30s most of should have a clear idea of what kind of metabolic rate we have:

- If you are highly active and losing weight is easy, you have a fast metabolic rate.
- If you enjoy moderate exercise and lose weight slowly, you have a moderate metabolic rate.
- If you don't enjoy exercise and find weight loss difficult, your metabolic rate is slow.

Figure 5

Height and Weight Chart (medium frame)				
Height (inches)	Normal Weight	Underweight	Overweight	Obese
57	102–133	101	134–150	151
58	104–136	103	137–153	154
59	107–140	106	141–157	158
60	108–142	107	143–159	160
61	111–145	110	146–164	165
62	114–149	113	150-168	169
63	116–152	115	153-172	173
64	119–156	118	157–176	177
65	122–160	121	161–180	181
66	124–163	123	164–184	185
67	127–167	126	168–188	189
68	130–170	129	171–192	193
69	133–174	132	175–196	197
70	135–178	134	179–200	201

Source: Metropolitan Life Height and Weight Tables

Whatever our metabolic rate, most of us feel less anxious if we are within the recommended weight ranges for our height. But height and weight charts like those in Figure 5 only give you a vague idea of your ideal weight for your height. They are typically based on mortality dates from people who buy life insurance, not disease and mortality statistics from the general population. These charts do not address the biological variability between women, such as how different our builds are, how our weight can fluctuate daily and with the seasons of the year, and how our bodies change with age.

Anorexia and Bulimia

Far too many of us in our 30s still believe that being thin keeps us looking young. Certainly too much body fat is an aging health risk, but if concern about appearance and fear of fat is taken to extremes, eating disorders can become far more of a threat to appearance and even life. There are women in their 30s who have conquered their eating disorders and look great because they now understand the basics of good nutrition, but there are also an alarming number of women who either continue destructive eating patterns from their 20s into their 30s, or who develop them for the first time.

Anorexia and bulimia can age a woman visibly and invisibly. The body is placed in a state of crisis. Without proper nourishment to the major organs, looks and health will suffer.

An anorexic tries to starve herself into a dangerously malnourished condition which she often hides with loose and baggy clothes. Even when very thin, she sees herself as overweight and is terrified of gaining weight. She is willing to sacrifice everything to stay thin, even the loss of youthful looks.

A bulimic binges on massive amounts of food and then vomits or uses laxatives or diuretics to purge her body. She may often go on strict diets and exercise obsessively. Bulimia is a secretive disorder. A woman may appear normal but maintains her weight with bizarre eating patterns. If the vomiting continues her stomach will begin to get distended. Her teeth will be like that of a much older woman because of the stomach acids that have worn away the enamel. Stomach and mouth ulcers are likely. Like an anorexic, hair, nails, teeth, and bones will suffer without the correct nutrients.

The problem is not usually cured by weight gain alone. Until a woman's emotional state is healed she can retain an anorexic mindset regardless of her body weight. Eating disorders often tend to occur and reoccur in times of stress. Frequently there is an unhappy childhood and poor self-image, and food obsession becomes a way to avoid dealing with unresolved emotional conflict.

Women with eating disorders need professional help and should make sure they get their doctor to refer them to a specialist or a counselor.

Borderline Eating Disorders

Full blown eating disorders like anorexia and bulimia tend to receive the most attention because of their shock value. For years now we have become used to hearing about anorexia and bulimia. Lost in the shuffle however are women with less severe cases of dysfunctional eating. "They don't take it so far but they hate their bodies just as much," says Joanne Stuart M.S., R.D., of Health Training Resources, a nutritional counseling firm in Branford, Connecticut (*Shape*, March 1998, p. 99).

Obsessive eating is defined by Frances Berg, editor of *Healthy Weight Journal*, in terms of how much time you spend thinking about food and weight. In *Afraid to Eat: Children and Teens in Weight Crisis* (Healthy Weight Publishing Network, 1997), Berg says women with eating disorders think about food 90 percent of the time. Dysfunctional eaters think about food 20 to 60 percent of the time. A poor body image is often combined with dysfunctional eating and obsessive exercising. These women exercise to burn calories, not to feel healthy. Their diets are dysfunctional in an effort to keep weight low, but not dangerously low. There is an irrational fear of gaining weight: "They base their happiness and their sense of self-worth on their food and exercise choices" (*Shape*, March 1998, p. 99).

Do you recognize yourself here? If you do then you fall into a category that professionals have trouble identifying, the shadowy world of borderline eating disorders. The condition is very common among thirtysomething women. You may not even know you have got it. Millions and millions of us obsess about our weight. We diet strictly. We exercise. We count calories. We get upset if we put on a few pounds. We think losing weight will make us look better, look younger. We wish we could lose weight. We feel more confident about ourselves if we lose weight.

Dysfunctional eating is dangerous and aging in the 30s. It could even develop into a full blown eating disorder. If you have poor eating habits and you exercise obsessively to lose weight, the costs to your health are high: nutritional injuries, bone loss, hormonal problems, injuries, and depression are likely. You probably won't lose much weight either as your body rebels with a sluggish metabolism. Without getting the nutrients you need you cannot expect to stay looking young.

The important thing is to get help if you are having problems with food and eating. You may need to get in touch with a doctor, counselor, or nutritionist.

Obesity

Being a little overweight doesn't seem to significantly affect our longevity, but being excessively overweight will. Almost any study on health shows that youthful looks and overeating do not go together. If you eat too much for your height and build on a regular basis and your activity levels are low, you will age far faster than someone who eats moderately and sensibly.

This is not to say that you should starve yourself, because there is no conclusive proof that a severely restricted diet increases life span, indeed a little bit of extra weight in mid-life and beyond has been shown to be beneficial. What is dangerous is not the occasional indulgence but indulgence on a regular basis which will eventually lead to obesity. Overeating puts a strain on your kidneys, liver, intestines, digestive system, and heart. Everything you do becomes tiring because of your weight, and you will feel and look older than you are.

If you can't control the amount of food you eat, you are suffering from a food addiction. It is crucial that you get in touch with a doctor, counselor, or nutritionist to get your eating habits back on track. Joining a support group may also help.

Weight Loss

Very few women in their 30s I talked to complained about being underweight. (If this is the case make sure you eat nutritious foods rather than junk foods to keep your weight up.) Most complained that as they got older they seemed to be gaining weight and this made them feel older.

In our 30s a weight gain of a few pounds often occurs naturally. Hormonal change, a more sedentary lifestyle, and a slower metabolic rate are all contributory factors. A few extra pounds won't do you any harm, but if you think you have weight to lose, following are a few tips about weight management in the 30s.

There are hundreds of programs to help you manage your weight. Some promise miracle results in short periods of time. Each of them has a different approach. The truth, though, is that no one solution will work for everyone. A method of weight loss that works for you won't work for someone else. You have to find what suits you. But if you want to lose weight there are four diet rules which always apply:

1. *Lose weight gradually.* Statistics prove that drastic weight loss is seldom effective and usually dangerous. Aim for loss of about a pound a week. A good weight loss program

ensures that you lose weight gradually and do not put it back on again when you stop.

2. *Increase your activity levels.* Basically, move about more. A regular program of exercise that includes aerobic, strengthening, and stretching exercise is best if you can manage it. If you lose weight by diet alone you will just look flabby and out of shape. Exercise gives you shape and tone. It helps your stomach and waist flatten and your hips look firmer. Exercise burns calories, but what is more important is that you build up muscle mass. Muscles burn calories more efficiently than fat. The more lean muscle tissue you have the higher your metabolism will be. The higher your metabolism, the faster you will lose weight and burn up fat stores.

   An exercise program for weight loss should include at least 45 minutes of aerobic exercise at least four times a week. Aerobic exercise means moving continuously for a period of time so that your body burns fat. You should be slightly out of breath but not so much that you can't continue a conversation when you exercise. To burn fat you also need to build up your muscle strength. Muscles need more energy than fat and burn up calories faster. Strength training needs to be a part of a weight loss program—and don't forget the importance of stretching and lengthening your body every time you start and finish your exercise routine.

3. *Eat to lose weight.* You need a balance of all the essential nutrients to feel healthy and to lose weight. If you want to lose weight, make sure your food intake contains all the nutrients your body needs.

   Diet for weight loss needs to be balanced and nutrient-rich. Eat less junk food and more healthy food. Losing weight safely and effectively is a matter of eating food that can boost our metabolism and burning up more energy than we use from our food. Foods rich in nutrients have magic properties that can eliminate hunger, erase water weight, and speed up your body's fat-burning power. The more nutrient rich foods you eat the slimmer you might get. You won't feel hungry all the time either.

On the other hand there are also foods that can interfere with metabolism and make you feel bloated and heavy. These include synthetic food additives, processed foods, foods high in salt, coffee, chocolate, and foods high in saturated fat and sugar. Try always to eat quality, wholesome foods free of additives and rich in nutrients. Avoid fast foods that are refined or processed or packed with sodium and synthetic additives. These kinds of foods don't have the substances you need for weight loss. Concentrate on whole, unrefined, and fresh foods rich in nutrients.

4. *Change your eating habits for life.* In order to lose weight permanently, you need to change your eating habits for the rest of your life. More fruits and vegetables, less fat and sugar, reduction in servings, and an adequate intake of nutrients are the best and most effective ways to lose weight.

Time and time again women in their 30s go on diets to lose weight and then put it all back on again. If you want to lose weight and keep it off, it is important not to go back to old eating habits. If you do, weight will pile back on again. Instead of dieting, think more of a permanent change in eating habits. From now on you are going to eat to maximize your chances of permanent weight loss, good health, and vitality.

Here are some other tips women in their 30s gave me about weight loss:

Throw Away the Scales

One of the best things you can do for yourself as far as weight management is concerned in your 30s is stop thinking about your weight and concentrate on how you feel, and trust your body to know what your natural weight should be. Hopefully the 30s will bring with them the wisdom and self-confidence you need to escape from what Christiane Northrup describes as the "diet mentality," when the number you read on the scale determines whether you have a good day and stands between you and how you experience your life (p. 576).

Sarah, age 33, says that she feels much better now that she has stopped weighing herself every morning. "At first I was scared because I thought I would lose control. But I didn't. Now when I hear other women talk about gaining or losing a few pounds I feel sorry for them. I was trapped like that once."

When you start to diet and go on your scales they will give you encouragement because initially you will lose water and glycogen from your muscles. You'll see a loss of a few pounds. But then next week, when you weigh yourself again, you haven't lost anymore. The same thing happens the following week and the scales demotivate you.

The reason you have stopped losing weight is because your body, fearing starvation, starts to cling to its fat stores. But this is, in fact, the most important time to keep going with your diet. You are close to losing weight but it will take time. That's why it's best to stay away from the scales which will demoralize you when you don't see any progress. Scales do not help you lose weight. They give unreliable and misleading information. Every day your weight fluctuates.

The scales don't tell you about emotional weight gain either when you have been eating poorly because you are sad or tired. "Don't rely on the scales to determine if you're successful or to provide you with a sense of self-accomplishment" writes Colleen Sundermeyer. "If you want to gain control over your eating and your body weight, get rid of the scale and listen to your feelings. You can trust yourself" (p. 26).

The best advice to give any woman in her 30s who is struggling with her weight is to stay away from the scale until you are emotionally ready for a weigh in—when the number on the scales has lost its power to determine whether you feel good or bad.

If you must have some kind of reference, a far better way to see if you are at a healthy weight is to ignore the weight charts and get your body fat tested. (Twenty-eight to 30 percent is normal. Under 25 percent is fit and slender. Lower than 22 percent is too thin. Higher than 30 percent is heavy.)

Stop Counting Calories

Many women who want to lose weight want to know how many calories a day they should be eating for weight loss. Statistics tell us that the average woman in her 30s is supposed to be eating around 2,200 calories a day. So if calories are restricted by 500 a day, a weight loss of 0.5 to 2 pounds a week can be expected, depending on activity levels.

No woman should consume less that 1,200 calories. Not only will this make you ill, if you are eating less than 1,200 calories a day you won't be getting the nutrients your body needs to stay healthy either. A very low calorie diet also won't make you lose weight. Our bodies have a Stone Age survival mechanism. If calorie intake is too low, metabolism slows down and fat stores are preserved for times of famine. Our body reacts primitively. It doesn't know that you are trying to lose weight.

Focusing on calories is not an effective way to manage your weight. "For five horrible years I was obsessed with calorie counting," says Anna, age 36. "I became an expert but I never seemed to lose weight." A reduction in the amount of calories you eat will help you lose weight but too much focus on calories can be frustrating. No two calories are the same. The calories you get from a banana are very different from the ones you get from a handful of sweets. Both might have the same number of calories, but the banana has more nutrient value. Making sure that your daily food intake is nutritionally sound. Getting nutrients in the right amount is a far more effective way to manage weight than calorie counting.

Rather than counting calories, it is far better to pay attention to your serving size. Even a few small reductions in serving size will make dramatic differences. You don't need to cut out your favorite dish, just reduce it, because eating too much is the most likely cause of weight gain. If you are trying to slim down, watch your portion size. For the grain group, for example, every slice of bread counts for one serving. The large bowl of spaghetti you had last week might have been as many as seven servings.

The standard portion sizes in the United States have been getting bigger and bigger. As a result, waistlines have gotten bigger too. If you follow the USDA food guide pyramid for serving size, you should be getting a balanced diet with all the vitamins and minerals you need.

- *Fats, oils, and sugar.* You don't need to cut these out entirely but you do need to eat them in moderation. It is fine to enjoy the odd chocolate doughnut. It is not fine to eat them every day.
- *Bread, rice, pasta, and cereal.* One serving is 1 slice of bread, 1 ounce of cereal, 1 cup of rice or pasta. The grain group gives you carbohydrates for energy, vitamins, minerals, and fiber. The recommendation is between 6 to 11 servings. If you are trying to lose weight, 6 to 7 servings might be right. High fiber foods, such as brown rice, are important in this group because they fill up and regulate your digestive system.
- *Vegetables.* Aim for at least 2 nutrient-rich servings, preferably more. One serving is $1/2$ cup of raw or cooked vegetables.
- *Fruit.* Aim for 4 nutrient-rich servings a day, preferably more. One serving is 1 piece of fruit.
- *Milk, cheese, and yogurt.* Two or 3 servings should be sufficient. One serving is about 2 ounces of cheese or 1 cup of milk.
- *Meat, fish, beans, eggs, nuts.* Two or 3 servings should be sufficient. One serving is about 3 ounces of meat or fish, 1 egg, or $1/2$ cup of beans.

Avoiding large portions means changing your routine to smaller more frequent snacks—around six meals a day, perhaps. This is because overeating at any one time overloads your system with sugar and fat. Fasting for too long slows metabolism. Most nutritionists agree that eating little and often are the most effective ways to lose weight and stay healthy. It is also important to eat your biggest meals in the morning and early afternoon rather than the evening when your body is preparing for sleep, not activity and digestion.

Change Your Eating Habits for Life

Not only does dieting not work because it fails to take into account the emotional reasons why we overeat, dieting also doesn't work because once dieting is stopped the old eating habits return. What is needed is a change in habits that lasts for the rest of your life. A whole new attitude to food that helps you maintain your ideal weight.

Body Basics

The real secret to successful weight loss seems to be making sense of all the conflicting advice out there. For every theory about weight loss there is bound to be one that says the opposite. But there are body basics you can rely on, the most important being that if you want to lose weight you have to exercise more, eat less, and preferably do both together.

Here's a review of the most helpful tips from women in their 30s who were successfully managing their weight.

1. *Keep as active as possible.*
2. *Combine strength training with aerobic activity.*
3. *Don't underestimate how much you are eating.* A food diary where you record everything you eat will be helpful. It is important to get an accurate sense of your food intake

and to watch your portion size if you want to lose weight.

4. *Don't go on restrictive diets.* Your body will cling to the fat if you do. You won't be getting all your nutrients, either.

5. *Don't get hung up on counting calories.* Make sure your diet contains a correct balance of all the essential nutrients. Concentrate on nutrient-rich foods that can help you lose weight.

6. *Don't cut out all the foods you enjoy from your diet.* You will only crave them and eventually succumb to a binge. Just eat them in moderation. Losing weight and being miserable don't have to be the same thing.

7. *The most effective way to lose weight is to do it gradually and slowly.* No more than a pound or so a week.

8. *Forgive yourself.* No one is perfect. So if you miss your usual workout or succumb to a cream mocha. Don't berate yourself and give up. Just acknowledge your slip—after all, you are human—and get back on track. It's what you do most of the time that matters.

9. *Stop weighing yourself.* Listen to your body and how it feels. Instead focusing on the scales, focus instead on exercise and eating right and feeling healthy. Permanent weight loss will follow along with other benefits: more energy, less aches and pains, and a good night's sleep.

10. *Be patient.* You will get there in time. And once you are down to your ideal weight make sure you continue eating sensibly and exercising so that the weight doesn't pile back on again.

Chapter 11
Taking Care of Yourself in Your 30s

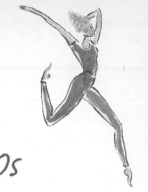

This chapter focuses on appropriate body care, makeup, and style in the 30s. It also stresses the importance of regular health checks and screening. Remember, though, that as far as body care is concerned, the place to start is not with a new skin care regime, or a new wardrobe, but with a new approach to your diet, exercise routine, and lifestyle.

This is not to say that skin and hair care aren't important. They are. The point is that no new hairstyle or chic outfit or nail polish will be able to help you look and feel your best if attention hasn't been paid to the basics: a healthy, balanced diet, exercise, and stress reduction. Without these foundation stones to delay the aging process you can't expect to feel energetic and vital. There is a direct correlation between what you eat and drink, your activity levels, and your stress levels with the health of your skin, hair, nails, and teeth.

My sources for the tips and advice given here are many and varied. I have learned from my own experience working in a fashion and beauty college and as a fitness consultant, from interviews with women in their 30s and 40s, from discussions with beauty and health professionals, and from extensive research into health, beauty, and antiaging secrets found in women's magazines, books, and videos.

Skin Care

If you want to age well you have to avoid overexposure to the sun and cigarette smoke. A lot of damage is already done to our skin by our 20s. Too much exposure to the sun unprotected by sunscreen will weaken collagen, causing premature sagging, and interfere with melanin production, generating age spots. It will also toughen the epidermis, causing a leathery texture to the surface of the skin; aggravate moles or beauty spots, making them potentially dangerous; and weaken the dermis layer, causing burst capillaries or spider veins. Smoking will cause wrinkles, give your skin a yellowy tinge, and make your skin look dry.

If you spent your 20s lying in the sun and chain-smoking, it doesn't mean that you will almost certainly wrinkle like a prune in your 30s. It will happen though, if you don't change your lifestyle now, in your 30s.

Taking better care of your skin in your 30s by avoiding the sun and stopping smoking will yield rich rewards. This doesn't mean you have to stay out of the sun altogether; it means getting used to using the key weapon against aging—sunscreen. Experts recommend that you wear at least factor 15 SPF all year round. Some dermatologists recommend 30 SPF to avoid wrinkling. Ideally it should be applied before you moisturize and given time to absorb before you put your makeup on. If you want that bronzed look in wintertime, avoid sunbeds. Sunbeds can accelerate the aging process faster than exposure to the sun. You might consider using bronzing powders or fake tanning creams.

Moisturizing daily or twice daily is also essential to protect the skin from environmental pollutants and keep it looking fresh and plump. Using the right kind of moisturizers that contain vitamins A, C, and E has been shown to thicken the skin. You might want to start thinking about applying moisturizer when your skin is damp to make it look less lined. A daily cream should prevent the skin from feeling dry, but it shouldn't be so greasy that it stops you from putting makeup on. A richer night cream should be used to boost nutrients and add extra oil to the skin. Avoid old-fashioned cold creams that are heavy and greasy and don't penetrate the skin. Better are the light modern creams, gels, and oils that are readily absorbed. It might be wise to avoid products with petroleum jelly and petroleum derivatives, as these can cause dry skin and other problems for some women. Important, too, is to keep your skin hydrated on the inside by drinking enough water.

Finding the right moisturizers might take time as your skin changes through the seasons and depending on how much time you spend indoors, outdoors, or in central heating. As well as moisturizing, you should spend time cleansing. Try to cleanse your skin twice a day to remove dead cells and to keep your skin healthy. Never sleep with your makeup on. This will clog your pores and cause blackheads and pimples. Make sure your cleansing routine is gentle. Skin cleansers come in countless forms from soap bars to creams. Regular bath soap bars can dry your skin, and clear glycerine soaps are too harsh. The older you get the gentler you need to be with your skin. Choose gentle cleansing soaps and if you decide to use toners make sure they are alcohol-free.

A skin specialist may recommend Retin A (retinoic acid), a form of vitamin A, for smoothing fine lines. Primarily intended for acne sufferers, Retin A can even out your skin texture and minimize lines, but it can cause skin irritation for some women. In many cases sunscreens work better than the much discussed retinoic acid, which is used by many women to retain their youthful complexion. Retinoic acid is available by prescription in a gel, lotion, or cream in a number of different strengths. After several months or years of regular use Retin A can undo some of the damage caused by the sun, but it cannot prevent further damage from occurring. It is a product that must be used indefinitely. It may also cause dryness, and there is concern that it might be linked to birth defects among babies born to women who used it during their pregnancy.

You might want to use alpha-hydroxy acid (AHA) cleanser or cream to slough off dead cells rather than exfoliators which can cause damage to your skin. Alpha-hydroxy acids are naturally occurring compounds that seem to be more forgiving than Retin A and have the added benefit of being available without prescription. Used regularly, they do seem to smooth the skin and some studies show that they also boost collagen production. If you decide to use AHAs avoid using them in combination with alkaline soaps; apply the cream to bare skin, leaving it on for about 10 minutes to be absorbed before using other products.

Other skin care products which are really moisturizers include antioxidants, which can protect against environmental toxins, and beta glucan, which is thought to promote a healthy glow. Ceramides and cerebrosides are natural components of sebum and good moisturizers. Collagen cuts down on water evaporation from the skin. Hyaluronic acid acts as a greaseless moisturizer, some believe liposomes keep the skin hydrated, and phospholipids keep the skin well moisturized.

As we get older the skin's ability to keep the outside world out and the inside world in is compromised and irritation and skin problems are likely. Gentle and restrained skin care can restore some kind of balance but the emphasis is on gentle and restrained. Choose your products carefully and remember that skin changes with time. You cannot always assume that your skin is normal. Aim to use products that are gentle on your skin. Avoid soap, scrubs, or anything that is too vicious. A gentle swipe with a washcloth, a weekly face mask, or the restrained use of a buf-puf-like sponge are all that is required to remove dead cells and brighten the complexion.

In general normal age changes to the skin in the 30s are minimal. To repeat, the main cause of changes in skin is not so much age but overexposure to the sun. Experiments have shown, in the words of Hayflick, that "sun truly ages the skin in ways detectable even at a cellular level" (p. 174). If you want your skin to stay looking fresh and wrinkle-free for as long as possible, wear high factor sunscreen all year long. The *Vogue* beauty experts agree and state that the sun is responsible for about 80 percent of the changes associated with age. "Deep wrinkling, sagging and bagging, leatheriness, visible blood vessels, sallow yellow coloring and brown spots are due to excessive sun exposure," according to the American Academy of Dermatologists (Hutton, p. 29).

When the sun hits the skin, free radicals are produced. These can go on the rampage and start to damage the skin. Fortunately the skin has a repair system, but even that is worn by repeated exposure to ultraviolet rays. Research is discovering that given time, the skin can heal itself if it is spared the onslaught of ultraviolet light. Harm caused by the sun is not irreversible, however, which must come as a comfort to all of you who spent your 20s sun worshipping. Research undertaken by the University of Pennsylvania suggests that conscientious use of sunscreen can undo some of the damage.

There is no real proof, though, that skin damaged by the sun can totally repair itself, so the message is clear. If you want your skin to stay looking young start wearing sun protection today, whatever age you are. This is especially necessary if you have pale, sun-sensitive skin, which ages much faster and carries a higher risk of skin cancer than tougher, darker skin. Choice of sunscreen is important. At present research is proving that a broad spectrum UVA plus UVB sunscreen is without any doubt the most important antiaging skincare measure there is. Make sure you check labels to see that UVA as well as UVB protection is included. This sunscreen should be applied everyday irrespective of the weather. Sunscreen contained in a moisturizer is fine as long as the SPF is 4 or more. An SPF of 15 is a bare minimum on sunny days; for prolonged exposure use higher SPFs, approximately 20 to 25. Needless to say it is wise to avoid sunbeds.

It's unlikely that in your 30s your skin will be so sun-damaged that creams and sunscreen can't reverse most of the process. If, however, you want faster, more dramatic results, there is the drastic measure of chemical peeling which literally burns away the damage and eliminates fine lines and wrinkles to allow fresh skin to grow. The problem with these kinds of procedures is that they often go wrong and they can be agonizingly painful. Another equally painful and controversial alternative is dermabrasion, which surgically removes the skin. Nonsurgical solutions for wrinkles include collagen injections, which act as a temporary solution until the next injection. Liposuction of fat in our thighs to our face is still in the realm of fantasy. Silicone seems to be the lesser of the line-filler evils but unless administered by a skilled expert the results can be disastrous. As far as sagging skin is concerned, for some women the only solution is plastic surgery, but this shouldn't be an option to consider in your 30s.

Most of us in our 30s, when we notice the first signs of dryness or wrinkles, tend to use more and more products and wear more and more makeup. Surveys show that the average American woman uses up to 20 products on her face everyday. But this could actually be making the problem worse. Sometimes less is more, and this is the case with skin. Use cream or oil to remove makeup. You may prefer soap and water but skip astringent toners—you don't need them. If you regularly use high SPF sunscreen this should help your skin moisturize again. If your skin feels irritated the first response is often to slap on creams and makeup. Such action, however, will only intensify the problem. The older you get the less you should be putting on your face and the more you should be leaving your skin alone. And what you do put on your face should be exactly right for it.

You can save your skin. Constant care makes all the difference. If you protect your skin all day long from the assault of ultraviolet light you can let your skin age at its own slow pace. If you start now you may be able to reverse some of the damage already done. However, taking an interest in your complexion does demand that you be realistic. In your 30s having great-looking skin doesn't mean having no lines at all. No amount of cream is going to recapture the freshness of youth. But if you look after your face in your 30s, it can look good in its own right. It will be more contoured and expressive and full of character. Take a look at some of the older models who model skin care products, like actress Isabella Rossellini or Andie MacDowell. Advertising companies are increasingly seeing faces that are beautiful because they have the look of maturity and experience.

Your Body

Don't forget about your neck and the rest of your body. The most visible signs of your age can appear on the neck. Skin on the neck is thin and vulnerable and if we extend our skin care routine to our neck in our 30s we will be doing ourselves a big favor. Cleanse and moisturize your neck daily and use night cream at night.

Use moisturizing lotion on the rest of your body too. You might also consider body brushing to remove dead cells. It can keep the skin soft and help work against toxin buildup, which can cause cellulite. Increasing your water intake will also keep your skin hydrated. Exfoliation, as long as it is not too harsh, can also help, as can occasional saunas and steams.

Cellulite. We all know what that is and in the words of Sharon Stone would "never trust" a woman without it. According to Elizabeth Dancey, author of *The Cellulite Solution* (1998), as we get older and our skin gets thinner our hormonally induced fat sacks get more visible. Women who work too much, who don't exercise, who eat poorly and drink too much often have more noticeable cellulite. There is no proven cure for cellulite and no magic cream to make it go away. The best thing you can do for yourself is to exercise regularly and eat well. Body brushing and keeping the area moisturized might help too.

Healthy Flying

Flying on a regular basis will dry out your skin. It puts a lot of strain on the system. You breathe in recycled air, and the atmosphere dries out your nasal passages, eyes, and skin, and has an aging effect whatever age you are. The lack of oxygen in the plane and the exposure to radiation make frequent flying a great health risk.

For many thirtysomethings frequent flying is an inevitable part of life. If you can, fly business or first class where the air is fresher, but if this isn't an option, sit as far forward in coach as possible. An aisle seat is better because it enables you to get up and down more frequently to prevent circulatory problems. Try to walk and stretch as much as possible. Avoid dehydrating alcohol on the plane and drink lots and lots of water. If you can, try to sleep for as much of the flight as possible and eat a very light meal. Bring eye drops to keep your eyes moist and lots of moisturizing face cream for your skin. Sit with your legs raised if you can and make sure you wear loose, comfortable clothes and shoes.

Foot Care

By the time we reach 30 all of us will have spent a day wearing shoes that make our feet sore. We will probably have also spent hours walking in high heels. We may not have lovely feet anymore. In our 30s our feet are beginning to lose some of their youthful padding. Skin gets drier, making them itchy, and poor circulation may cause swelling. You may notice clumps of hard skin or calluses, or start suffering from foot problems like ingrown toe nails and athlete's foot. Nothing can make you feel older than painful feet. They stop you from being as active as you want to be.

The 30s are a good time to start looking after your feet. Chiropodists are not just for older people, but for people of all ages. Good foot hygiene and health will keep you feeling youthful.

The most important thing you can do for yourself is give your feet good support and structure with well fitting shoes. As the soles of your feet begin to wear down, support them by adding cushy inner soles to your shoes. Make sure that all the shoes you wear for each activity are properly fitted by a shoe professional. If you have worn high heels for years you may notice that your Achilles tendon has shortened, making walking barefoot uncomfortable. If you have worn shoes that are too tight you may suffer from bunions, blisters, and corns, which can not only make older feet uncomfortable, but unattractive too. As we age our feet do become slightly broader and longer. Don't keep wearing the same shoe size you always have. Get the size that is right for you.

If you have swollen feet this is probably due to circulation problems and standing and sitting too long in one place. Swollen ankles and feet can really look ugly. They can be a symptom of heart disease or lymphatic problems, so make sure you get checked out by a doctor. They might also be caused by the equally unpleasant vascular problem called varicose veins. Varicose veins are caused by—and also cause—poor circulation as the blood tries to return against the force of gravity to the heart through clogged vessels.

If you have circulation problems there is a lot you can do yourself as well as checking with your doctor. Keep moving whenever you can. Avoid sitting and standing for long periods of time. Avoid crossing your legs. If the problem is with veins sit with your legs raised when you can but if in doubt keep your legs on a stool to raise your thighs to improve circulation. Investing in a good pair of support stockings may help, as can evening primrose oil and sessions with a reflexologist.

It is rare but women in their 30s can and do get bunions. Bunions are the painful outgrowths of bone matter on the inner side of the foot near the big toe. These painful developments not only hurt but cause swelling too. Usually bunions are inherited by women who have a big toe that curves toward the other toes instead of growing straight. It is probable that this nasty condition is caused by wearing shoes that are ill-fitted and too tight.

If you have a bunion or two wear shoes that are made of natural fibers and are not man made. Make sure they are properly fitted. Try to correct foot rolling by investing in specially molded insoles. You can get orthotics by prescription from an orthopedist. In the last resort an operation to straighten the bunion may be necessary but as they can sometimes be unsuccessful it is perhaps better to try and prevent bunions reaching such an advanced stage when there is no other alternative.

If you have corns and calluses your shoes don't fit correctly so invest in a pair of properly fitted shoes. You can treat corns and calluses with an emery board when dry and then moisturizing after they have been softened by warm water. Ingrown toenails hurt a lot. To prevent them buy shoes that give your toes room to move when you walk. Cut nails straight across to prevent the nail growing in. If you do have an ingrown toenail, see a specialist for treatment and don't try to dig them out yourself.

Those who have smelly feet may have a fungal problem which can be treated by sprays, or if the problem is persistent, by a doctor. Use antiperspirant on your feet to prevent your feet from getting damp and sticky. Wear shoes and socks made from natural fibers that give your feet room to "breathe" and expand. Remember, feet are at their largest at the end of the day so this is the best time to do your shoe buying.

Feet should be washed and dried daily and rough, hard skin removed with a file. Frequent application of moisturizer will guard against cracking. Toenails should be cut straight across. As they thicken with age they may need regular attention. Monthly pedicures are not an indulgence. Remember, in the words of Goethe, that a pretty foot is something beautiful that defies age.

Norman Orentreich of the Orentreich Foundation for the Advancement of Science in New York and his colleagues have found that from the age of about 30 fingernail growth slows by around 50 percent. Most changes that occur in fingernails, like dullness, color change, and splitting are normal, but some dermatologists believe they may be due to excessive exposure to the sun or to nutritional, temperature, or hormonal effects. Toenails, on the other hand, don't seem to change much. Their growth rate remains constant.

Hand Care

Hands convey so much about a woman. In your 30s you may notice that your hands start to resemble your mother's hands. You could notice more prominent veins. If hands and nails have not been taken care of they can at times be embarrassing. Too much hot and cold water, detergents, sunshine, and wind can make your hands look worn and dry. Skin may be peeling and nails cracked and the hands lined. Faces have natural oil but hands don't have their own so if you haven't been moisturizing them or putting sunscreen on them or wearing rubber gloves for washing up, your hands won't look that good.

Hands, like a woman's neck, can give away her age. Hands convey much about a woman and the kind of life she leads. Hands that aren't cared for can make even a beautiful woman look unattractive. Lovely hands are the result of genetics, lifestyle, and diet. We can't do much about the first, but we can do something about the others. Good nutrition is evident in the strength and color of the nails. White flecks show zinc deficiency and dryness and ridges can mean not enough B vitamin. Healthy nails should be pink. Weak nails may also be due to lack of calcium.

The basics of good hand care are obvious. Avoid hot and cold liquids and detergents, and protect them from sunshine and cold weather. Try to use rubber gloves whenever you can. If you use your hands a lot and are a potter, a painter, a cook, a craftswoman, and so on, extra care needs to be paid to your hands.

By our 30s, nails will be more likely to splinter or break; they may also be thicker and drier. Diet is particularly crucial for the length, look, and appearance of nails. Anything that benefits the nails will also benefit the hair, discussed in the following section. Particularly important nutrients are vitamins A, B, C, and E; zinc; calcium; iodine; sulfur; and iron. Biotin, found in eggs, may also be a useful nutrient.

Homeopaths and Ayurvedic practitioners can read the state of your health from your nails. Nail ridges might start to appear and they, like rings on a tree, can be a sure way to age you and show up the state of your health. Some homemade solutions can effectively strengthen nails, like soaking them in warm olive oil or cider vinegar.

If you use nail polish, short nails tend to be more manageable. Applying a base coat and a top coat will prevent chipping. Don't cut cuticles or pull hangnails, and avoid sawing back and forth when you use an emery board. Filing nails in one direction will prevent splitting.

Nail color can make hands look particularly well groomed but not if nail polish is applied badly. The secret is to use good products and not to hurry, giving the nails plenty of time to dry. Some nail polishes contain strengthening agents which are particularly good for weak and brittle nails. Don't go overboard on nail polish though; it is important that every few months you let your nails breathe and be exposed to daylight. Nail extensions should be avoided because they weaken and damage your nails.

Hair Care

Hair comes low in the list of priorities as far as the body is concerned. This means it often misses out when supplies are scarce. Because of this, the look of your hair is actually an excellent indicator of your general health. If hair looks lank and flat and color changes it is highly likely that nutritional deficiencies are the case. Excessive dieting and skipping meals can tell on the hair's condition, thickness, and shine, because they deprive the hair follicles of the nourishment they need. It may take several months for hair condition to improve if diet is poor, since it takes a while for the old hair to grow out and new hair to appear.

Decades ago, once women reached their 20s their hairstyle remained constant and never changed. Things have changed now. A new hairstyle is the fastest way to change your image and how you feel about yourself. The biggest challenge is finding a stylist whom you can trust to give you a style that suits you and not them. Hairdressers are notorious for making assumptions about what their clients want without really considering the shape of their face, character, or build. Once you find a stylist you feel comfortable with try to get a trim every six weeks or so to keep split ends at bay and the hair well conditioned.

There is no one way to wear your hair in the 30s. You have to find what makes you feel good. Just don't expect the same hairstyle you had in the 20s to look as charming now. Your hair changes as you get older and gets a little thinner and will need extra care and attention. In general when I spoke to stylists they preferred shorter hair on women over 30. Short hair all of one length can show off the neckline and shape of the head. Many women in their 30s do take the plunge and "graduate" from long hair to short hair, and have been amazed at the difference it makes. They feel much more confident, as if their faces have transformed. Short hair is a sign of self-assurance, confidence, and of having grown up. A short hairstyle never goes out of fashion. It is also the most practical for a woman with a busy life.

According to stylists, long hair works best if you are in your teens. Long hair in the 30s can be aging, but then again long hair can look amazing on some older women. There are exceptions to every style rule, and you may be one of them. Jane Seymour and Jerry Hall, for instance, have made long hair at mid-life glamorous again.

Gels, mousse, sprays, and the new styling aids now available from hairdressers offer the ideal solution for women who have hair that is difficult to manage. It is important, though, that you know how to use these products correctly and remember that often less is more. Overapplication of mousse or gel can make hair look flat. Use the smallest amount—about the size of a grape.

Regardless of whether or not you notice the odd gray hair or two in your 30s you will soon discover that hair needs managing in a whole new way. What worked before may not work now or look so good. Your hair just looks, feels, and behaves differently than it did in the 20s.

As we get older, hair tends to get dryer and more frizzy because the activity of the sebaceous glands slows down and the supply of sebum, a natural oil which keeps the hair looking shiny, falls off. When the cuticle loses its protection, moisture evaporates. Various things the hair is exposed to, like shampooing, blow-drying, waving, coloring, and ultraviolet light, can make the situation worse by lifting the cuticle. Hair looks worse.

Once hair condition has gotten worse, paying too much attention to your hair may actually make it worse still. Once the cuticle has lifted it will soak up whatever you give it and no conditioner will improve how it looks—in fact it may make it worse. Overconditioning hair is one of the main reasons hair looks dull and lank. Women find themselves in a vicious cycle. The worse their hair gets the more products they put on it and the buildup continues. The answer is to use a gentle shampoo and to rinse thoroughly afterwards. An acid rinse may be preferable to a conditioner. Add the juice of a lemon to some water. Rinsing is very important for your hair to look in good condition; that's why at the hairdresser's there are usually so many rinses. If your hair is very lanky try a shampoo, like Neutrogena, that doesn't contain any conditioners at all.

Take special care of your hair when it is wet, as it loses its elasticity. Any further pulling caused by brushing, combing, or excessive toweling could make it snap. When blow-drying try to ensure that hair is already half dry. Dry downwards to keep the cuticle flat and keep the dryer on the move constantly so that you don't overdry. If you must use styling tools, like heated curlers or rollers, try to restrict their use to once a week. Heated rollers can boost a style, but they can also damage the hair if used excessively.

In our 30s every hair on our head has a growing phase that lasts nearly three and a half years, and a resting phase of three months before it falls out. About 150 hairs should be shed every day but after three decades hair spends more and more time being idle and less time growing. Hair doesn't usually get noticeably thinner until the 50s, but some women in their 30s do suffer from thinning hair or even balding, which might be due to hormonal imbalance. If this is the case hormonal therapy may be a solution. Using natural products on your hair, avoiding rough treatment, and eating a nutritious diet might help. Nutritionists recommend an adequate intake of biotin, found in oats, soybeans, brown rice, and green peas, which is needed for healthy skin and hair.

Many women in their 30s start to color their hair. This could be to keep the gray at bay or to give their hair a new vibrancy, with either highlights enhancing their natural hair color or a complete color change. Highlighting or lowlighting protects the scalp from contact with the dye, and if you are at all worried about the health risks of hair dyes, they are safer. There is no conclusive proof, but certain cancers have been linked to the use of permanent and semi-permanent hair dyes. If you have the odd gray hair, highlights, lowlights, or vegetable conditioning colors that have a lower concentration of chemicals are the best option.

If you plan to color your hair yourself, choose a well known brand like Clairol or L'Oréal, and remember that treated hair needs extra care and maintenance. Choose shampoos and conditioners with neutral to acid pH such as those labeled pH-balanced or containing citrus fruit, milk, or beer. If you are considering curling your hair, find a skilled operator. If you go out in the sun for any length of time, make sure you protect your hair with a leave-in conditioner, a hat, or a water-soluble hair sunscreen, as ultraviolet light can shorten color-expectancy and lighten the color quickly.

Teeth

Thanks to new developments in modern dentistry, there is no reason why anyone should have unattractive teeth. We should be able to keep our own teeth well into old age, but tooth decay is still a problem because few of us seem to find the time for proper oral hygiene and too many of us eat too much sugar. Sugar's destructive corrosiveness causes gum disease. If gum disease causes the gums to recede to a point where the roots of teeth are exposed, they become vulnerable to decay.

Gum disease, when bacteria can become trapped in the gum line and ultimately erode the bone that holds teeth fast in the jaw, is like many of the problems associated with old age—preventable. With proper dental care, a good diet, and regular checks, virtually all of us can prevent tooth decay.

Brushing and flossing at least twice daily is essential because it removes plaque from on and between our teeth. Plaque is a mix of food debris, skin cells, and bacteria that continually collects in our mouths. If it is not brushed or flossed off within 24 hours the mineral in saliva will start to calcify and within a short time set into hard tartar which can only be scraped off by an oral hygienist.

Most of us brush up and down and back and forth but this is inefficient and fails to get into all the hard-to-clean corners. This heavy handed approach also wears down the enamel on the front surface, which can cause tooth sensitivity. The best way to brush your teeth is to brush at a 45 degree angle and to wiggle the brush against the teeth so the bristles poke in between. Each tooth must be brushed with care and the whole process should not be rushed. Toothbrushes should have small heads (about the size of a child's toothbrush) to be most effective in removing plaque. Most brushes are far too big. Bristles should be medium or medium-soft and toothbrushes changed as soon as the bristles begin to fan out. Brushing should be followed by flossing. Floss around the teeth in a C shape and sweep up and down. Use floss rather than toothpicks, which are not as flexible.

According to Dr. Michael F. Roizen of RealAge.com, flossing and brushing will keep you looking younger longer. Gum disease can lead to aging of the circulatory and immune systems and daily flossing and brushing can knock a good five years off your biological age (your age according to how healthy your body is) as opposed to your chronological age (how old you actually are).

As long as the right toothbrushing and flossing is employed and plaque removed every day, the bacteria in plaque is rendered harmless. If tooth care is inefficient, however, plaque can change the nature of your teeth. Bacteria delve into the gums, causing redness, inflammation, and bleeding on brushing. Bleeding gums are always the first sign that all is not well. The American Dental Association has estimated that by the age of 35, three-quarters of all Americans have signs of gum disease—namely bleeding, inflamed, and receding gums—but are unaware of it. If gum disease is not checked, teeth will become loose and abscesses will appear.

If you want to keep your teeth well into old age, proper dental hygiene in your 30s is essential. New research has shown that gum disease is already well advanced in many women in their 30s, although teeth won't fall out until later. Regular visits to the dentist are essential for everyone—twice a year is recommended, and more if there are problems. In the early stages, regular scaling of hardened tartar and root planing, which scrapes away bacterial deposits below the gum line, can keep the disease in check, but once it reaches a certain stage even the best dental hygienist can do very little.

It is not just gums that change with age, teeth do too. Wear and tear and food additives can yellow them, flatten them, and make them more brittle and likely to chip. Increasingly, cosmetic dentistry is turning its attention to supplying clients with younger looking teeth or attempting to realign problem teeth. The pearly whites of Hollywood film stars are becoming possible for others—but at a price.

Makeup

> *I glanced in the mock Victorian pub mirror. I looked like a garish clown with bright pink cheeks, two dead crows for eyes, and the bulk of the white cliffs of Dover smeared underneath. Suddenly I understood how old women end up wandering around over-made-up with everyone sniggering at them and resolved not to snigger any more. . . . I'm prematurely aging.* (Bridget Jones's Diary, p. 147)

Since your skin and its coloring are changing in your 30s you may need to rethink your approach to makeup. What worked well years ago may now look tired and heavy and dated. Techniques and color selections used can announce your age before you open your mouth. In your 20s you could get away with wearing too much makeup. Less is certainly more as the years get better. Wearing too much makeup Barbara Cartland style can be, as Bridget Jones found out, aging. The colors we used to wear may no longer be suitable. In your 30s you might find yourself cutting down on the amount of makeup you wear.

When it comes to makeup you shouldn't need to spend hours applying it. Ten minutes is more than enough. Too much makeup can look unnatural and aging. It's not good for your skin either. If you don't wear any makeup, make sure that you use sunscreen and moisturizer to protect your skin. If you do wear makeup, the first thing to do is to clear away all the clutter in your makeup bag and choose only colors that complement your looks as they are now. You may need advice from a makeup specialist here.

Light diffusing foundation is good for making lines less noticeable. Trying brands that also offer protection from the sun is advisable. If you choose to use a concealer to even out darker areas on your skin, avoid those that are so light they look chalky and unnatural. Translucent powder will give you a light matte finish. Use upward strokes when you apply your blusher. For best effects use a lighter color on the cheekbone and a deeper color underneath. Avoid brown blushes, which can look aging.

Eye shadow, eyeliner, and mascara can give thirtysomething eyes more definition. Use upward strokes when applying eye shadow and be careful not to drag the corner of the eye. Eyeliner all around the eyes, however, tends to make them look smaller. Color under the eyes tends to accentuate lines and wrinkles. If you use eye shadow, harmonize it with your eye color. Brown or hazel eyes look best with soft, brown shadows; blue or gray eyes are heightened by gray mixed with another color. Mascara can be applied last in a thin coat. Curling the lashes before the mascara may open up and lift the eyes. Eyebrows and lips often thin with age—pencilling with colors will fill them in. Don't draw a line if you use a pencil, since this can be aging; use soft strokes instead. Applying your lipstick with a brush gives a lighter, even stroke than applying it directly from the stick. A natural lip pencil to outline the lips as well as to fill them in may make lips look fuller. Remember to choose your lip color wisely. Some colors, like orange, can make aging teeth look ugly.

Makeup should not dominate your morning routine. Think of it as something to enhance your best qualities. The goal is not to let people see your makeup first but to see you and how special you are.

Style

"In your thirties, you can get away with just about anything provided you are fit (and not flabby) and have the personality to carry it off" (Spillane and McKee, p. 280).

In your 30s you can enjoy experimenting with a variety of styles provided you take care of your body and have the right personality to match. We shouldn't have to worry yet about how short a skirt should be, how flared is flare, and whether see-through blouses are appropriate or not. There will probably be the odd item or two in our wardrobe, like those platform shoes or leather miniskirts, that we feel faintly ridiculous in, but on the whole the 30s should be the decade when we try to have fun with fashion.

There aren't really any fashion do's and don'ts. But remember that how you dress announces to the world what kind of a woman you are. We have all seen those films when the secretary who wears gray suits and spectacles and a bun suddenly transforms into a glamour queen when she changes her image, lets her hair down, gets contact lenses and a designer dress. Frumpy clothes can be aging whatever stage in life you are in, and the 30s are no exception.

The same suit you wore to your first interview six years ago may have gotten you the job, but wearing it now that you have gotten a promotion may not work since you want people to view you differently. A new look doesn't have to mean a whole new wardrobe. It just means getting out of your rut and dressing in the way that makes you feel good and that projects the image of yourself you want to project. Have a look through your wardrobe and pick out a few of your favorite outfits. Think about what your objectives are in life and whether your clothes match up. Get rid of those clothes you never wear or can't fit into anymore. Rethink what you have left to make you look how you want to look.

"Nothing is sadder or more frightening than seeing a woman of the more interesting age in clothes too girlish or revealing. It makes her appear as if she is out of touch with herself. And she is" (Hutton, p. 110). Aim to build up a wardrobe that reflects who you are and what you want to express at this stage in your life. Do the colors you wear really flatter you? Does your makeup fit your outfits? Think about the accessories you wear. Most fashion editors of magazines are in their 30s so you might find it useful to look at trends and suggestions there. Keep reviewing your wardrobe. You will look older than you are if you get in a fashion rut.

Remember anything goes concerning fashion in the 30s, but only if you take care of your body. You won't look good in miniskirts if you are flabby. If you are fit and toned, clothes will just look better regardless of how so-called perfect your shape is. If you want to look slimmer avoid details and clutter on your clothes, gathered waistbands on skirts and trousers, and busy patterns, and avoid tops and jackets ending at the widest point. Bring attention to your face by opening up the neck area, wear clothes that fall straight and elegant shoes. Shorter haircuts that frame the face and lift from the side and back are also slimming.

Looking at yourself in a full length mirror can be helpful. See what you like and what you don't like about your outfit. But if you know you find it hard to be really objective about yourself you might find it useful to ask friends or better still an image consultant. A good image consultant should be able to help you look and feel good about yourself. They cost money but if you are lucky you will receive some advice that will last you a long time.

Hopefully this is the decade when we find our own style voice so that when mid-life comes we can dress eloquently and make fashion work for us. We all know women who took several decades to find their sense of style and who look a million times better in their 30s or 40s or 50s than they did in their 20s, such as Lady Diana and Jackie Onassis.

Medical Screening

We have big advantages over our mothers and grandmothers as far as health is concerned. We are more educated about our bodies and screening offers an unparalleled opportunity to catch problems before they become aging or life threatening. Regular checkups can ward off cancer, heart disease, osteoporosis, diabetes, and blindness. Screening can also help us make appropriate health choices and determine whether or not we need to change our lifestyle and have more regular checkups.

Following is a list of screenings most relevant to women in their 30s. Bear in mind though that screening techniques are not always perfect and that new research is developing all the time which may make our current screenings and blood tests seem inaccurate and clumsy.

- *Blood pressure.* Take at least once every two years and more often if you are on the pill, overweight, a diabetic, or you smoke. This is to check for hypertension, a recognized factor in heart disease, stroke, and other health problems. Moderate changes in blood pressure can be brought down by lifestyle changes rather than drugs.
- *Blood/fat analysis.* Every five years, to measure total and HDL cholesterol. High cholesterol may contribute to the development of heart disease, especially if other risk factors like smoking or being overweight are present. A high result should provide the motive for lifestyle changes.
- *Blood glucose.* All women in their 30s should be aware of the warning signs, which include fatigue, extreme thirst, blurred vision, frequent urination, and persistent infections, such as cystitis and yeast infection. Many women who suffer

from glucose intolerance are not aware that they have the condition. Regular checkups are advisable. If you think you may have a problem, there are reliable self-tests over the counter; or talk to your doctor and ask for a glucose tolerance test. Women who are at high risk (family history of diabetes, sugar in their urine, gestational diabetes when pregnant) should be especially vigilant.

- *Bones.* Women at high risk (those with eating disorders or who exercise intensively or who have hormonal problems) should consider getting a bone scan for osteoporosis.
- *Breasts.* Clinical examinations by a doctor or a nurse once a year to pick up breast cancer as soon as possible so that it can be taken out and is less likely to spread.
- *Cervix.* A pap smear test every year to pick up possible cancerous changes in the lining of the womb which can be permanently obliterated by laser before they become dangerous.
- *Colon.* Women at high risk (bleeding from the colon, a history of colon cancer in the family, marked change in bowel habit, abdominal pain, weight loss) should take a yearly fecal occult blood test, which can detect changes which one day might develop into cancer.
- *Eyes.* Regular eye tests at your optician every one to two years can catch early changes. Eyestrain can be avoided by prescribing the correct lenses for your eyes and early changes corrected which might damage the eyes. Individuals with a family history of glaucoma should be screened every year from the age of 35. Diabetics and hypertensive individuals may need more frequent checkups.

Taking Responsibility for Your Health

If your doctor doesn't take any of your health concerns seriously find a doctor who does. Proper health care and preventative medicine in your 30s could make the difference between looking and feeling years older than you are and looking and feeling healthy, vital, and energetic.

Finding a sympathetic doctor and feeling able to talk about health issues that concern us is all part of taking greater responsibility for our health. The 30s are the decade when we start realizing that our bodies have limits. Unless we start treating them right, they won't perform optimally. Much of our health and well-being is in our hands.

American nutritionists now say that we have two ages: our chronological age—that is, how many birthdays we have had—and our real age, which is the actual age of our bodies according to how well we have taken care of them. Studies have shown, time and time again, that women who eat a healthy diet, exercise regularly, avoid alcohol, cigarettes, too much sun, and too much stress, have a real age considerably younger than their chronological age. So if you are worried that you might in fact be years older than your birth certificate, that you might be 35 going on 45, that your body is aging faster than you are, it's up to you to start taking responsibility for your health now.

Chapter 12
Enjoying Life

Enjoying your life is important if you want to lead a fulfilled and satisfied life. The 30s can be a busy decade as far as work, social life,
and family commitments are concerned. Many of us are eager to prove
ourselves and make our mark, but in the process we may neglect to
also enjoy ourselves. Remember the saying, all work and no play
makes Jill an unhappy woman. And being unhappy or feeling stressed
accelerates the aging processes faster.

Think about all the things you really enjoy doing and then think
about trying to work as many of them as practically possible into
your daily life. Research is now proving that pleasure does the
immune system good. The more fun you have the more gracefully
you will age and the healthier you will feel. When we are happy,
positive hormone and enzyme levels are elevated and blood pressure is normal. When we are unhappy, stressed, or anxious, levels
are lower. Even smiling can send impulses along the pleasure
pathway to make you feel good. And besides, wrinkles from smiling
are far more attractive than harsh frown lines.

Many studies have linked happiness to longevity and demonstrated that there are considerable health benefits in happiness and
good humor. From the interviews I conducted it soon became
apparent that positive thoughts keep women looking and feeling
young more than creams and lotions and surgery. Not only is it
important to find pleasure in your daily routine, but to keep planning ones in the future.

If you don't have enjoyment in your life, if you don't have love, laughter, and fun, then are you really living? One thing is sure—you won't feel or look as healthy as those that do enjoy life.

Rethinking Your Definition of Attractiveness

"Every woman knows that, regardless of all other achievements, she is a failure if she is not beautiful," writes Germain Greer in *The Whole Woman* (1999, p. 19). And beauty in today's culture means being thin, tall, and young.

As the great majority of us in our 30s are not tall and thin it's not surprising that millions of us hate our bodies. Body hatred has reached epidemic proportions in the last few decades. An industry has sprung up and made billions from the fact that American women hate their bodies. Diet centers, plastic surgeons, fitness centers, and weight loss clinics are everywhere. We all, it seems, want to be thin, tall, and young. We want to look like the scrawny models who parade on the catwalks and hold before us an impossible ideal to aspire to.

One of the biggest stumbling blocks many women in their 30s face when it comes to enjoying life is a poor body image. Feeling unattractive stops us from living life to the fullest. Body image insecurity tends to be a feature of the 20s, but for millions of women in lingers on to haunt the 30s. It affects every aspect of our lives and is a major cause of fear, anxiety, and depression.

A poor body image has a great impact on all areas of your life. According to Thomas Cash, Ph.D., of Old Dominion University, body image constitutes a huge 25 to 33 percent of a person's sense of confidence. A poor body image can contribute to depression, low self-esteem, and obsession about your physical flaws, all of which are aging. It uses up energy that could better be used for creativity, productivity, and self-realization, according to Marcia Germaine Hutchinson, a Boston psychologist and author of *Transforming Body Image* and *Learning to Love the Body You Have* (1997). Body hatred can also damage your health and may even lead to stringent dieting and obsessive exercising that can contribute to the development of poor health or disorders such as compulsive eating, obesity, anorexia, or bulimia.

Body hatred is unattractive at any age. So what do you do if, like millions of other women in their 30s, you are not only worried about the early signs of aging but you hate the way you look? What do you do if you don't feel beautiful?

The chances are that if you begin taking care of your body with the right diet and regular exercise you will start to respect and like your body more. But this won't happen overnight. In the meantime you have to stop trying to change your appearance and start trying to change the way you feel about how you look. Changing the way you think about yourself won't be easy. Be patient with yourself and give yourself time. Take consolation from the fact that you are not alone and that you have to fight years of conditioning in the wrong direction.

Here are a few tips from women in their 30s which might help.

- Being thin, it seems, does not improve your body image. I spoke to many women who had lost fat or who were at or below their ideal weight who still disliked their bodies.
- Spend some time really looking at other women your age. Notice how very different their bodies are from each other. What makes one woman attractive may make another look unattractive. Think about people you consider beautiful. Often their features are not perfect.
- If you think you are overweight get your body fat tested to see if you fall within the normal range. Twenty-two to 25 percent means you are relatively slender and physically fit. If you are athletic 28 to 30 percent is okay.
- Get to know your body better. Have a look at yourself naked in front of a mirror. Counteract negative thoughts about your body with something positive. Instead of "I look fat," focus on how beautiful your eyes are, how good your hair looks,

how great you look in a certain color.

- Have a good long think about why you want to look different. Why is it so important to you?
- Do some research. In many cultures around the world being thin is not considered attractive. The men of Matsingenka, a remote tribe in Peru, for instance, have a fixed standard of beauty very different from ours. Shown pictures of western models the men grimaced and announced that the women must have diarrhea. They approved instead of women with no waists and layers of fat. Also, in times past the idea of beauty was far from thin. There was a time when the cultural standard of beauty was plump. The so-called "Venus de Willendorf" female body type dominated the imagination of the known world for 25,000 years as archeological finds from Iceland to Mongolia confirm. The woman with excessive fat, especially in the buttocks, was admired in Rubens's day, when famine and disease still reigned. Remind yourself that today's ideal of beauty is a cultural construction.
- Listen to your body. Commit to trusting that it knows what it wants. Be honest about what you are eating. Make sensible, healthy food choices. Eat when you are hungry. Stop when you are full. Exercise when you can. Not only will this aid weight loss but it will boost body confidence.
- If how you look is really making you depressed, seek professional help. You need guidance about how to change negative thought patterns, and a therapist might help. Call an eating disorder clinic at your hospital and ask for a referral. To keep you on track you might consider joining a support group that deals with food, weight, and depression.
- Read some books on developing a healthy body image and self-esteem. A good place to start would be *The Beauty Myth: How Images of Beauty Are Used Against Women* by Naomi Wolf (1992).
- Try to identify the real triggers for your body hatred. Every

time you feel negative about your body think about what is going on at the time. Are you really angry with your husband? Has your boss upset you? Did you feel ignored by the shop clerk?

- Recognize that it is unnatural and unhealthy to look like the models on the catwalk. They are not representative of real women, but fantasies created by the media.
- Understand that thinness and youth do not equal attractiveness.
- Separate what you do from how you look.
- Focus on what you are good at. Put your energy into other things. Focus on other areas of your life.
- Most important, remember that a positive body image makes a woman attractive regardless of her build or weight. Gaining this kind of body confidence starts with treating your body with respect.

Hopefully in our 30s we will have realized that whether we have long legs, short legs, a large build, or a delicate one, we will nonetheless get older. We should have moved beyond the desire to appease a youth obsessed culture. We should have understood that it is time to rethink our definition of attractiveness. Beauty is not about youth and slenderness but about feeling confident about ourselves as women. It is not about how slim you are, how big your breasts are, and how young you are, but about self-awareness, self-satisfaction, and a positive body image. And the sooner a woman comes to this realization the happier she will be. The less she will mourn the passing of her youth and the more she will look forward to the years ahead of her and all challenges and opportunities they bring.

Enjoying Your Work

Pleasure does not have to be separate from work. The ideal scenario would be that you found work that gave you a sense of vocation or pleasure—that you loved what you did for a living. There is nothing more aging than watching the hours tick by at work, day in and day out. Being a workaholic is not the same as being someone who is enthusiastic about her work. The latter often find that her life is so invigorating that she rarely need vacations. The former is driven and obsessed, a woman who doesn't have time for anything meaningful.

Being happy in your work means enjoying it as part of a balanced life. Research shows that if you have a sense of control over what you are doing at work you often enjoy it more. This doesn't mean taking over the organization. It means taking initiative, organizing your routines as much as possible. If your job doesn't allow you this freedom perhaps you should think about another working environment.

Some job advertisements might cause you concern in your 30s. Those that legally can't specify race or sex can still ask for candidates under the age of 35, for example. Age discrimination in your 30s can and does happen, but never let any employer convince you that you are too old to learn a new skill or trade. The real reason some employers favor teenagers and youth has nothing to do with age. It has to do with budget. Younger people can be paid less. Decline in working skills is not inevitable as you get older. You will probably be able to organize your schedule better and prioritize. Plus you have the added bonus of experience and maturity. According to Malcolm Hodkinson, former professor of geriatric medicine at University College of London, "We experience a series of tradeoffs as we get older: experience and skill can trade off against physical abilities" (Spillane and McKee, p. 296).

Don't become the stereotype as you get older and stop learning new skills at work. It is often assumed that the older you get the less able you will be to adapt to changing circumstances. As your body starts to age, don't let your mindset follow suit. You may get the odd wrinkle or two, but you don't have to be inflexible. The ability to be flexible, to adapt to change, is the distinguishing feature of women who age successfully. These women think life is a big adventure.

They move with the times, not just in work, but in all areas of their lives. They stay current, interested in the world around them. They don't live in the past. They aren't backward looking. Look at how Madonna has changed her image over the decades. She is as sharp now as she has ever been, but had she continued to dress in her "Into the Groove" style she would have long been forgotten.

Your mindset, not your chronological age, is what can hold you back. So take advantage of every opportunity that is offered to you. Keep pace with what is current. Continue to learn. Keep up with the gossip. Find yourself a mentor to inspire you. Stay in the mainstream. Don't fall into the trap of thinking that it's easier for older men to be high profile at work. A recent study showed that women who work in their mid-40s enjoy higher self-esteem and more job satisfaction than younger women. This is the decade when women are promoted to higher level positions, and as the years go by their success is consolidated. Life at work really does begin at 45 if you rise to the challenge.

Image is important at work, especially if you are in a position of authority. Don't let your image fade in your 30s; keep it current and look the part. Take note of efforts to sideline you; make sure what you have to say is heard and that your opinion is taken into account. Use body language and eye contact to get your point across.

And if you don't work, make sure that you love the life choices you have made. That you have friends, interests, hobbies, hopes, and dreams. People who love what they are doing tend to look younger. If you don't really enjoy your life and have at the moment no avenue of escape because of financial or family commitments, for your own sake find an interest that really motivates you. The important thing is to make the most of every day of your life. And if work is a large part of your life you owe it to yourself to ensure that you use every day as an opportunity to learn, to grow, to be challenged, and to enjoy.

Stop Comparing Yourself with Others Your Age

"Just as certain mood enhancing drugs make a girl sensitive to the sunlight, turning 30 will make her ultrasenstive to the accomplishments of everyone else." (Tilsner, p. 89)

Comparing yourself with others is one sure route to unhappiness. It's natural of course because we all have expectations of what we should be, what we should have accomplished and many of us may feel that we have fallen short. And in every area of our life where we feel we have let ourselves down there will be others our own age who have succeeded.

In this modern age of young whiz kids, it can be hard not to feel that you are lagging behind. But however beautiful, successful, and talented your best friend is she will have anxieties of her own too. And there will always be women who are better than you in some things. That's just a simple fact of life. Don't attend school reunions if they are going to depress you, and try to avoid reading or hearing about those more successful than you.

Concentrate on your life, your skills, your talents, and what makes you unique.

Let Go

Just because you were best friends at school does not mean that you have to dutifully keep in touch when you have both grown apart. Just because you have trained for a career does not mean you have to stick with it when you not longer feel fulfilled by it.

A major part of the maturing process is recognizing when it is important to let go. Relationships, mindsets, and careers that suited you in the 20s may not be appropriate now and could even be stopping you from maturing. This doesn't mean you have to abandon all that was a part of your life in the 20s, it just means having the maturity, courage, and insight to recognize when to stay committed because it is still enriching and when it is time to move on.

Be Independent. Be Yourself.

Hopefully in your 30s maturity and self-confidence will gradually replace a vulnerable need for the approval of others. You are not so afraid to stand out in the crowd. Somehow it doesn't matter so much anymore what others think. The important thing is whether or not you are being true to yourself. You discover that you don't always need friends, parents, or partners to validate your every action and thought. That you begin to enjoy your own company and trust your own opinions. Expect to find this scary at first, but in time having the courage to be yourself and think your own thoughts is one of the most truly wonderful gifts that the 30s bring.

Positive Thinking

Positive thoughts will keep you looking young and enjoying life. The sooner you come to the realization that time is precious and that all the time can be quality time the happier you will be. Always seeing the negative instead of enjoying the moment and looking forward in anticipation to the future will only lead to depression and frustration which are aging states of mind.

Being negative about everything implies that you are also fearful, anxious, resentful, and stressed. That you are one of those people who sees problems instead of solutions, who says "I can't" instead of "I will."

This is not to say that you should agree to everything. For some of us with poor self-esteem learning to say "no" and not feel guilty is an important step to make. Learning to be more assertive, to value your own opinions, and be less influenced by the opinions of others, is a major rite of passage in the 30s. It is simply to say that in the

30s being negative all the time is unhealthy. Being more positive is vitalizing. If life has let you down, it may at times be hard to develop a positive mindset, but an upbeat approach to life really is crucial for feeling and looking youthful.

Trying to be more optimistic and less pessimistic is a technique that can be learned. The next time your notice yourself reacting negatively to something, check yourself and see if you can see the positive side of things. If you can't summon up any enthusiasm for something, if you feel constantly bored, if something beautiful, like a painting or a song, doesn't give you pleasure, if you have no interest in the future, you may be very depressed. It is important that you seek medical advice immediately.

Caught halfway between the resilience of youth which can keep depression at bay, and the maturity of midlife, which can help you deal with it, women in their 30s seem to suffer from depression more than any other age group. There are as many causes of depression as there are women who have it. Perhaps we have reached a point when what we have achieved with our lives so far doesn't match up to all to our youthful expectations of life. There may be some kind of addiction or compulsive behavior. Or we may be under great stress at work and at home. We could have suffered a loss or experienced a traumatic event. Then again there could be hormonal imbalance or even a chemical imbalance in the brain. Nutritional deficiencies could be the problem as could lack of exercise and sleep. Whatever the cause, depression brings with it extreme tiredness, changes in sleep pattern, irritability, problems with eating, and loss of interest in life. It is aging.

Diet could play a key role when your mood is low. Fresh green, yellow, and orange vegetables and fruit can help lift your spirits. Dairy and wheat products as well as alcohol, caffeine, and too much junk food can aggravate them. Depressed people also seem to respond positively to nutritional supplements of vitamin C, vitamin B complex, calcium, magnesium, zinc, and folic acid. Depression can also be triggered during the winter months when serotonin levels are low due to the lack of sunlight. During the winter months light boxes with full-spectrum light may be helpful.

Feeling down is not necessarily a symptom of depression, but if the mood is persistent it is important to seek the advice of a medical expert. If clinical depression is diagnosed you need the support and care of your doctor.

Expressing Ourselves

We may be frightened of negative emotions, and indeed emotions like anger, fear, worry, and sadness can be stressful. But the expression of our emotions, including the negative ones, is important for our physical and mental health. This is not to say that we should act on them all the time, but we should acknowledge that these emotions exist in order to alert us to areas of discomfort in our lives. Stifling our emotions will cause even more stress. When they are bottled up they affect our whole body, especially the immune system, because we are not allowing ourselves to feel and act as we should.

Scientists are only beginning to understand why crying has a soothing effect. It appears that crying is the body's way of washing out stress hormones. So when people say they are crying it out this is literally what they are doing. Stress is linked to an increased risk of poor health, and since women cry more than men this could be one of the reasons we live longer.

Crying and laughing, feeling and expressing our emotions is natural and human and very different from depression, negativity, and bitterness, which are unhealthy states of mind. Suppressing or not acknowledging our emotions can be unhealthy because our emotions are the only real way that we have to acknowledge that our life matters to us. Feeling our emotions shows us how important our life is to us and how important it should be to those around us. Sometimes these emotions will cause us pain and distress, but negative emotions also signal the need for some kind of change in our lives. They require us to act, to change the situation that is causing distress, to rebel against what we see as an injustice, to move on with our lives. Negative emotions are not always bad emotions, they can be necessary for us to grow and develop. The only bad emotion is one that is not acknowledged.

Wicked Pleasures

In moderation, many guilty pleasures, like eating chocolate or drinking a glass of wine, won't do us much harm. But you have to have been living underground if you have not heard about the health risks of cigarette smoking or alcohol. Certainly, enjoying ourselves is good, but not if guilt is involved. I would guess that there are very few women in their 30s who smoke or drink excessively without the guilty knowledge that what they are doing isn't good for them. If so-called pleasures make us feel guilty and unhealthy, they aren't good for us anymore.

It's necessary to distinguish between treating yourself and being addicted to a substance. Having two cookies and enjoying them with a cappuccino is very different from eating the whole pack and drinking four cappuccinos. There is a great difference between an afternoon at the mall doing some retail therapy to a shopaholic's addiction.

You will find that pleasurable activities are comforting and make you feel satisfied but that addictions are usually avoidance habits and they don't leave you feeling comforted. True pleasures are not the same as feeding addictions. Pleasurable activities, like going for a bike ride or visiting the beach, produce endorphins or pleasure enzymes which are good for the body and make you feel good. Other so-called pleasures like smoking or drinking are not good for your body and won't make you feel so good. It is important to appreciate the difference. You will know the difference if you are in tune with your body and listen to the signals it sends you. Are you hungry or just bored? Do you really want that drink, or do you want to forget the argument that just happened? Do you need a cigarette, or is it because you don't know what to do with your hands?

If you treat your body right and listen to its messages it will treat you right as well. Ignore it and there will be conflict between your needs and your body's needs, and this will manifest in wrinkles, flabbiness, and dry skin.

Friendships

Good friends and happy partnerships can really help you enjoy your life. A close circle of friends can make a big difference. Studies have shown that loneliness and isolation can be prematurely aging.

Whether you are in a relationship or not, thirtysomething girl-friends can help you realize that you are not alone. That you shouldn't panic if you haven't done all the things the magazines say you should and shouldn't have done by the time you are 30. No doubt your friends will have their anxieties and fears too, and there is nothing more therapeutic than a bit of good advice or a group bitching session with friends who are going through the same thing as you.

Friends can help you keep calm about being 30, give you a sense of perspective, and make life much more fun.

Keep Learning

You may finish school or college, but the school of life is never finished. You need never stop learning and growing as a human being.

There can be such pressure in the 30s to settle down, get that house, get that promotion, and have those kids that life can all too often stop you from challenging and developing yourself. It is easy to fall into the trap of thinking that you know all there is to know, that you have grown out of the student phase. But unless you want to prematurely age, being an eternal student will keep you young and current. Stay interested in what is going on in the world and what the current trends are. Learn about things you didn't know anything about. Learn not for where it will lead you but for learning's sake. If you can do that you will not only feel vibrant and youthful but you will be a pleasure for other people of all ages to know.

Always remember that it's never to late to learn anything you want to.

Keep Laughing and Playing

Children laugh hundreds of times a day. Women in their 30s probably only laugh about 50 times a day. If just the act of smiling can produce demonstratively lower stress levels, think what laughter can do. When you are stressed or anxious, your sense of humor is the first thing to go. A shared sense of humor is what keeps relationships together.

Being in your 30s does not mean you suddenly have to become serious. Being serious and responsible are not one and the same thing. Laughter is cathartic. Find time for it in your busy life and never mind that your pelvic floor isn't what it used to be.

There are also health benefits for playing. Playing shouldn't stop just because you aren't a child anymore. As well as being great time-outs, using your imagination or playing imaginative games can benefit concentration, coordination, attention span, and general health and well-being.

Stay Sensual

The act of sex itself is a health bonus. It can be a good form of exercise, stimulate the pleasure centers of the brain, be a stress reliever, and release human growth hormone. Orgasm, whether it is achieved with or without a partner, sets off a chain of positive neurochemical reactions that should leave you feeling rejuvenated.

Don't ever feel that because you have cellulite and your breasts aren't quite as perky as before that you are any less desirable. Stay sensual and you will have what Dr. Michael Perring calls a "moist look" (Spillane and McKee, p. 392). Sensual people don't tend to look dried up. There is always that sparkle in their eye. You may have a partner to keep sensuality in your life, but if you prefer to stay single make sure that you are surrounded by good friends and treat yourself to sensual pleasures, like a massage or a bubble bath, regularly.

Finally . . .

At the end of the day remember that however well you eat, however regularly you exercise, and however much weight you have lost, if you don't enjoy your life you won't feel good. A life without enjoyment, full of stress, anxiety, and fear won't be kind to you as the years go by. It will age you fast.

PART FOUR
EVERYONE AGES

"The age of a woman doesn't mean a thing.
The best tunes are played on the oldest fiddles."

—Sigmund Z. Engel

•   •   •

"To know how to grow old is the master work of wisdom and one of the most difficult chapters in the great war of living."

—Henri Frédéric Amiel

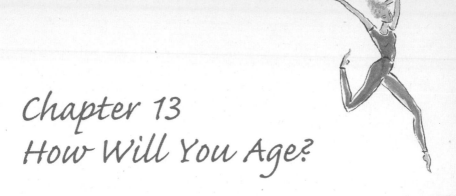

Chapter 13
How Will You Age?

Here's what Jill, age 36, thinks about her age 30 transition.

"Looking back I think turning thirty was an exciting time. A lot has changed for me in the last five years. I look more grown up. I like the respect I get. I like the fact that I have some experience of life. I like not being at the bottom of the ladder anymore. I like being a woman. As far as my body is concerned I feel very happy with it. I take care of it. My curves don't bother me anymore. In fact I quite like them. They announce to the world that I am a woman."

Moira, age 35, is not quite so upbeat. She has mixed feelings.

"Some days I feel really positive but other times I get really anxious. I never really thought about life over thirty. I don't feel thirty-five at all, whatever thirty-five is supposed to feel like. I like being more mature but I'm scared of being ill, of looking old and frail, and of losing my independence. There is still so much I want to do but a part of me says I'm too old to start something new. Some days I would give anything to be eighteen again."

Monica, unlike Moira and Jill, prefers not to think about aging at all.

"I don't want to think about it. I don't want to think about getting older." It does upset Monica that her friends seem to be settling down, that they seem to be growing up faster than she is, but underneath it all she thinks they still envy her freedom. She dates men years younger than she is and is never short of an invite to a party. To live this fast lifestyle she has to work hard to look young. She exercises two hours a day and barely eats to maintain her sylph-like figure. So far she has avoided wrinkles but she says she wouldn't hesitate to have plastic surgery or hormone injections to maintain her youthful allure. "Everything in life is competitive," she says. "Looking young is no exception. If you are too lazy to work on yourself you can't expect to look good. I can't imagine a time when I will ever give up and grow old without a struggle."

Sarah, age 37, has also decided not to think about aging. But her approach is at the opposite end of the coping-with-age spectrum. "I just don't bother much about how I look anymore. Aging is a fact of life. I can't fight it. So I may as well enjoy myself. I eat what I want, drink what I want. And I'm dammed if I'm going to stop smoking."

Monica, Moira, Jill, and Sarah represent varying points of view in the how-to-deal-with-aging processes. Jill is fiercely positive about it all, Moira is not so sure, Monica is in denial, and Sarah has just given up.

If you are like the majority of us in your 30s you probably recognize a bit of yourself in each of them. Some days you feel on top of the world, reveling in your newfound maturity. Other days you may feel anxious. Then comes that day when you decide to lose 10 pounds, have a new haircut, and make a commitment to work out daily. And then there are the times when you think, "To hell with it all. I just can't be bothered anymore."

Whatever your approach, how well you cope with getting older depends largely on how well you cope with life in general and how well you can accept reality. In your 20s you may have been able to avoid dealing with life's harsher side, but in your 30s sooner or later you are going to have to deal with the reality of getting older. There will be times when you feel negative and anxious. There will be times when you feel sad. There will be times when you don't think you can cope. This is normal. You are not age-phobic or in denial, just a woman coping with change. Change is challenging and invigorating, but it can also be scary.

"Little did I know that the transition from being a 20s girl to a 30s woman would be so dramatic," says Sue, age 35. Sue admits that the transition was unsettling. That she was relieved not to feel 30 on her thirtieth birthday. And her biggest fear was physical change.

"To be honest, I didn't notice any real change till I hit thirty-two. I recall the anxiety of being twenty-nine. Bad habits were formed in that one year; nail biting, yo-yo dieting, and chasing the wrong kind of man. And all because the dreaded thirty was looming and I didn't know how I should be. (As it happens my thirtieth birthday was spent in bed sick with a dose of flu. I felt good though, tucked up in bed like a nine-year-old. Bliss. My dream had come true—I didn't feel thirty at all.)"

Sue finds that she studies herself more these days. "I now see those tiny lines that form at the top corners of the mouth. Were they always there, I ask myself? Perhaps it's just that I never noticed them before. I stand for ages at the bathroom mirror examining my face inch by inch. I pull faces and try to determine where the next line will appear. I've even been known to share a joke with myself, throwing my head back in mock raucous laughter before the punch line to determine what I must look like to others. The lines are definitely there mocking me as though I'm the last one to get the joke. But this isn't a joke. It's not funny."

A fitness enthusiast, Sue recalls how she could exercise for hours at a time day after day in her 20s. "Not the case now, I hasten to add. Energy, now there's a funny thing. Now you feel it now you don't. Where does one's energy go? Always been accustomed to expending high energy through sport. I never experienced a problem with my energy levels. Then I hit 32—wham! I noticed in that year that an hour's session would feel like an eternity. I would jump and twist and turn and enjoy giving my all but that would last for the first twenty minutes. I'd then hit a plateau in my energy output and my enjoyment would end. The last forty minutes would become a battle of wills—how can I conserve my energy and still keep up with everyone else. The trick is smaller movement, edge your way to the back of the class and keep smiling."

But at the end of the day Sue is enjoying her life. She tells us that being in her thirties isn't all doom and gloom. "Despite my fear of change, I am actually having a ball." She tells us that the 30s are "a chance to really get to know yourself better. To be wiser, more confident, more self-assured. To be good to yourself. To enjoy yourself. A time of true self-discovery. You can explore your body, explore your mind. It's exciting. You can be selfish or be generous. You can be you. Some days I have more energy and on the days I don't I use my wisdom to overcome it."

Getting older is an attitude thing. You can approach it in a relaxed, humorous, positive manner, like Sue is, or you can go into denial, like Monica, and try to fight the process every step of the way. But the end result of trying to unnaturally prolong a youth that has passed away can only be depression and frustration. Far better to deal with the inevitability of change by taking the best possible care of yourself and accepting that with every loss there are always gains and changes. Although you are leaving your youth behind, you are entering a new and exciting phase of life where the old rules don't apply anymore. What worked when you were in your 20s may not be appropriate now. Your life is moving on and you need to change with it.

Being in your 30s changes everything. How you feel, how you think, and maybe even how you look. Your twentysomething years won't ever come back, but if you are patient and treat yourself with respect you will find in time that this change is for the better. Don't think that coming to terms with this change is the same as giving up. Nothing could be further from the truth. If this book has taught you one thing hopefully it will be that getting older has nothing to do with giving up, illness, stagnation, and depression and that it has everything to do with good health, constant change, and vitality.

But, whether or not it is entirely depends on you. Expect to feel anxious about getting older. This is normal. Remember that what counts in the end is how you choose to lead your life. How you choose to age.

Aging in the Future

In the future there may indeed be magic formulas for delaying the aging process. The most brilliant minds are applying themselves to the question of why and how we age and in the new millennium amazing conclusions may be drawn from current studies. At present, research into human DNA is making the science fiction of our dreams become the reality of our lives. Already we can have babies-to-be screened against certain illnesses. For instance, a gene for baldness has been discovered. Genes for cancer may soon be located.

It is possible that all of the diseases associated with aging that we might get could be wiped out in the womb. It is conceivable that one day scientists will be able to turn off the clock that is genetically programmed to cause our cells to self-destruct after a number of divisions. Regeneration of human body parts is already becoming a distinct possibility, as are Ova banks where women can deposit their healthy young eggs for use when they feel ready to have a baby. Antiaging specialists seem determined to redefine our allotted time span to at least 120 years. Amino acid supplements and human growth hormone injections supervised by a specialist are being offered at antiaging clinics. Antiaging cosmetics are also becoming more readily available.

How we age in the future may be very different from how we age today. But, despite all the incredible advances, antiaging experts are still grappling with the same eternal questions. Is aging a natural process or a disease? Is modern science tinkering with the natural order of things? What are the implications of a world full of people over 100? In our lifetime we won't know the answers to these questions. All we do know at present is that certain things can accelerate the aging process and avoiding them not only promotes longevity but improves quality of life at the same time. We also know that the younger you are when you start taking better care of yourself the greater your chances of looking and feeling vital. There are great health benefits to starting a healthy lifestyle program in your 40s, 50s, 60s, 70s, and beyond, but taking care of yourself in your 30s really is the optimum time.

Aging, like life itself, will probably always remain a mystery. But for now, and maybe till the end of time, the recipe for successful aging stays the same. It is all about good genes, luck, a healthy diet, regular exercise, absorbing work and interests, love and laughter and being positive. You can't change the good gene and good luck part. But you can do something about the rest, and this book has shown you how. If you take responsibility for your mental and physical health in your 30s, the quality of your life now and in the decades to follow will certainly and dramatically improve.

One Day

In our 30s when time begins to show itself on our faces and bodies, in spite of the huge change in society's perception of women in their 30s, 40s, and 50s, we may still be mystified and shocked by our own aging. It can be hard for our self-image to adjust to the fact that we aren't young anymore. We may be jolted into the recognition that we are aging by a sudden illness or the death of a friend or parent. We may catch a glimpse of ourselves in the mirror to see an image which seems different. Aging and bodily flaws begin to disgust us. We may pine for those days when we could take our appearances for granted.

We may panic and try to beat the clock. The age of face lifts is dropping and many women are starting to have them in their 30s in an attempt to retain their youthful appearance rather than recapture it in mid-life. But sooner or later all of us have to come to terms with the fact that we can't stay 29 forever, however much we would like to and however much money we spend on ourselves. Whatever we do age happens, whether we like it or not.

Apart from the loss of youthful looks there are other changes and losses to face in the 30s. Physical change always accompanies mental and emotional change. There may be the realization that our life plans and youthful ambitions may not ever be realized, that our present strivings may not be as meaningful as we would like, that we are not as mature as we had hoped we would be. That we haven't done all we think we should have done.

Adjusting to the loss of our youth can be like mourning a death. There can be shock and disbelief followed by denial, anger, and resentment, but if there is a recognition that getting older also brings gains and new insights, the desire to stay forever young can seem like ultimate denial.

The psychoanalyst/social psychologist Joan Raphael-Leff notes that many women spend their early adult years waiting for that "one day," that magical moment when everything will fall into place. When their real life will begin. The subtle signs of aging in the 30s bring with them the realization that at least a third of your life is over. That "one day" may actually be here. This can be a difficult time, but it has its positive side. It can stop a woman from spending her life in preparation or rehearsal. She may start living every moment more fully in the present. She cares less—not doesn't care—about what others think of her. Instead of postponing things, she realizes that there isn't necessarily going to be a "later." She seizes the day.

It's good to be aware of the fact that we are aging. The knowledge that one day our lives will end isn't as depressing as it sounds. It keeps us alert to the truth of our lives. And that truth is not about looking forever young but about being a woman with a changing body whose life will one day end. Thinking about that end might be frightening, but knowing that our lives and our bodies are finite brings clarity to every decision we make. That's why the prospect of immortality is seldom comforting except to antiaging scientists.

Awareness of our own mortality gives our lives a sense of urgency without which we would probably lack motivation to do anything. It helps us know what is in our best interests. It helps us respect and value what is uniquely our own. It helps us understand that the "one day" we dreamed of is now. There is no point holding back waiting for something magical to happen and our lives to fall into place. It's up to us to make the magic happen now. Not just the 30s, but the rest of our lives are about taking responsibility for our lives and how we age, about constantly reinventing ourselves, about constantly learning about ourselves, and about living each day as fully and as vitally as we possibly can. About seizing the day.

There is life after 20. Women do not go insane at menopause and get depressed in old age. Evidence is growing that the older a woman gets the more content and robust she is, the higher her self-esteem and sense of fulfillment. In fact, women who consent to leaving their youth behind and enjoy being their age can escape from the insecurities of the 20s and find freedom from the tyranny of youth and prettiness. Getting to that place can be liberating and empow-ering. Many women in mid-life marvel at how strong, wise, resilient, and aware they feel simply because they are older. As the final chapter shows, many of them wouldn't want to be 20 again, when they felt no sense of their own power.

Chapter 14
The Prime of Your Life

Once we start seeing the 30s as a time that can deliver us from the insecurities and uncertainties of the 20s rather than a time of loss, the crisis softens. "Once in a while all the old insecurities come back," says Julia, age 33. "I'm trying on clothes in a changing room and I wish I was more toned and younger looking. But most of the time I really don't care what others think. Life's too short."

The 30s are a decade of transition, physically, mentally, and emotionally. You leave girlhood behind and become a woman. Don't expect it to be smooth sailing all the way as you notice the subtle signs of aging. Crossing over to the 30s is a time of crisis, and times of crisis are never easy to handle. But the way we deal with all the crises, challenges, and obstacles life presents us shapes our personalities, helps us understand who we are and what we want out of life, helps us grow up.

Sometimes in the midst of the thirtysomething crisis it can be hard to see the light at the end of the tunnel, to get a sense of perspective. So in the process of writing this book I talked to women who had successfully navigated their way through to the other side. Women in their 40s. The message was overwhelmingly positive in almost all cases. It was perfectly natural to feel anxious about leaving the 20s behind. In time the anxiety would go. The 30s really were the beginning of the prime of your life.

This Is My Life

Many women who have gone through the turning 30 crisis wondered what all the fuss was about. They didn't feel that much different. It was all a bit of an anticlimax. "I remember waking up and thinking, Is this it? A bit like the first time I had sex. Life just goes on. You don't look or feel that much different," says Joyce, age 48. Linda, age 40, says that when she hit 30 she actually felt a lot younger than she thought she would. It wasn't the huge turning point she expected it to be.

After relief that the world hadn't collapsed and they didn't transform into old women overnight, many women said that they experienced a different feeling. They felt a bit stronger. Being 30 gave them more confidence, which made them look and feel better than ever before. And this newfound confidence was a trigger to evaluate exactly what was happening in their lives. The transition from childhood to adulthood brought focus and an overwhelming sense of individual responsibility. Helena, age 42, found that coming to terms with this new responsibility was liberating. "Everything became much simpler. I stopped waiting for things to happen to me. I realized that this was my life and that I was responsible for it. If I wasn't happy only I could do something to change that. I ended my relationship and started a whole new career in publishing."

Margaret, age 40, also found this sense of responsibility, but for her leaving the 20s behind was all about letting go of values, experiences, and even people that belonged to the 20s. "Getting older has made me less fixed in my ways. Turning thirty brought me the wisdom that you can't hold on to things or people. Life is about constant change. At every stage in your life you redefine yourself. In my twenties, I thought that the people I mixed with, what I thought, and what I did would be always the same."

Rachel, age 49, realized in her 30s that she had options. That she could create the circumstances of her life. "It's strange, when you are young, you think about the thirties as this time of conformity, but looking back I can see that I was far more conformist in my teens and twenties. I wanted to be part of the crowd. To fit in. Now I want to stand out from the crowd. Have my own opinions. Do my own thing."

It became clear to me from my conversations with older women, that the 30s, rather than being a time of panic because we hadn't done all we thought we should, are about learning from our past. We are old enough to learn from our mistakes but young enough to start something new. We start to assess our priorities. This doesn't mean that we alter dramatically as we leave the 20s behind but that certain things in our lives start to change.

Hopefully we get a clearer picture of who we are and what we want out of work, family, friends, partners, and from life itself. We know what we don't want to do as far as work is concerned and what we won't put up with in our relationships. We become more discriminating. "It dawned on me," says Amanda, age 41, "that I had choice. I didn't have to keep going out with the same group of people. I didn't have to stay in the same job. I could make changes."

Part of having a clearer picture of who we are and taking responsibility for our lives is the new respect many women have for their bodies. Ann, age 40, says that she actually has a better body image now that she had in her 20s. She started to appreciate what she had rather than lament what she hadn't. "I'm enjoying my body. I'm tired of trying to look a certain way. Now I enjoy looking like me. If people have issues with my weight that's their problem, not mine."

Along with greater confidence we can also discover a new sense of self-respect and honesty. We are more true to ourselves, which involves not blaming yourself for everything, realizing that you are not the center of the wheel, that how people behave and what people think is their problem, not yours. So the 30s are about being more centered in yourself, in knowing who you are and what you want. You realize that how other people feel and act is not your responsibility.

Deborah, age 41, says that in her 30s being honest with herself involved identifying herself less with externals and becoming more focused on how she felt about herself. "I realized that if I was ever going to be happy I had to stop only feeling fulfilled if I was doing well at work or in a relationship. The 30s taught me how to be alone and to be happy in my own company without it being validated by things or people. It was such a relief."

Life Begins at 30

"Whatever a woman does, she must not age" writes Germaine Greer in her 1999 polemical text *The Whole Woman* (p. 22). But when I talked to "aging women" the message did not tend to be one of regret, depression, and longing for what was. The 30s were not the low point that marked the beginning of decline. In fact, they marked the beginning of empowerment, freedom, and change.

Empowerment means that you feel more certain of yourself as a person. A negative comment won't send you into floods of tears anymore. You begin to really understand that beauty is far more than skin deep. That it's impossible to look good in a convincing way if you aren't sure of yourself as a woman. Freedom means that you realize you have choices. Just because your mom always said you would be a great mother doesn't mean you have to have kids. The possibility of change means that you realize that decisions you made in the 20s can be altered. That life is about constant change and adjustment. That life is a voyage of self-discovery.

If we can learn self-respect, a sense of balance, a sense of personal integrity, and openness to change, the 30s will indeed be a time of great accomplishment. Don't panic if you are in your 30s and you still feel confused, anxious, and trapped rather than empowered, liberated, and free. This is all part of the process of growing up, learning about yourself and your strengths and weaknesses. The 30s can be a painful time. It can be hard to see a way forward when you are in crisis. Hopefully these words of inspiration from older women will give you the courage and strength you need to deal with the pain and crisis.

Feelings of crisis and confusion are an essential part of life if you are to grow as an individual. Without crisis there would be no change and when there is no change there is only stagnation and decline. Crisis points continually appear in our lives to help us explore our full potential. When we are stagnating they force us to ask questions about who we are and what we really want.

And don't think that if you make it through the crisis of turning 30 you won't have any crises again. Life is a constant series of crises. Being able to respond to crisis points in our lives, make adjustments, change course, and reinvent ourselves is what keeps us vital. And hopefully as we get older and gain in maturity and experience, life will give us the wisdom, flexibility, and openness to the new things we need to cope with each new crisis and period of change.

All this emphasis on crisis and change doesn't mean that as the years pass we won't recognize ourselves. Our identity will undergo change but there will always be a certain continuity. Women in their 40s and 50s told me that the 30s were really about gaining deeper, richer self-knowledge about making sense of their lives. "Now I'm in my sixties," says Margaret, age 65, "I look back and as bizarre as it sounds there is a strange pattern to it all. Nothing I ever did was wasted. Even those things I thought at the time were not right for me. It taught me something and became a part of me and my life."

Ageless Beauty

Finally, talking to women of all ages about getting older made it abundantly clear to me that getting older has nothing to do with becoming less attractive. A positive body image and self-respect are what makes a woman attractive—regardless of her age and how much cellulite she has.

In your 30s everything that mother nature gave you, father time will start to take away. But our changing bodies can encourage us to become more knowledgeable about ourselves so that we maximize our beauty, fitness, and vitality well into old age. If we can accept the reality of change gracefully and really start listening to our bodies, then aging in the 30s can become something more than feeling old or listing bodily complaints or trying to look young enough for a youth-obsessed culture. It will instead be about self-satisfaction through self-acceptance and self-awareness. It will be about looking in a mirror and liking what we see.

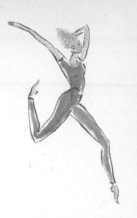

Suggested Reading

Borysenko, Joan. *Minding the Body, Mending the Mind.* Bantam, New York, 1987.

——. *A Woman's Book of Life: The Biology, Psychology and Spirituality of the Feminine Life Cycle.* Riverhead, New York, 1996.

Brumberg, Joan Jacobs. *The Body Project: An Intimate History of American Girls.* Vintage, New York, 1997.

Chernin, Kim. *The Hungry Self: Women, Eating and Identity.* Harper Perennial, New York, 1994.

Clegg, E. M. and S. Swartz. *Goodbye Good Girl: Letting Go of the Rules and Taking Back Yourself.* New Harbinger, Oakland, California, 1991.

Claflin, Edward, ed. *Age Protectors: Stop Aging Now.* Prevention Health Books, Rodale Press, Inc., Emmaus, Pennsylvania, 1998.

Dancey, Elizabeth. *The Cellulite Solution.* St. Martin's Press, New York, 1997.

de Beauvoir, Simone. *The Second Sex.* Vintage, New York, 1952.

Dietrich, Edward B. and C. Cohan. *Women and Heart Disease: What You Can Do to Stop the Number One Killer of American Women.* Times Books, New York, 1992.

DiMona, L. and C. Herndon. *The 1995 Information Please Women's Sourcebook: Resources and Information to Use Every Day.* Houghton Mifflin, New York, 1994.

Dockett, Lauren and Kristin Beck. *Facing 30: Women Talk about Constructing a Real Life and Other Scary Rites of Passage.* New Harbinger, Oakland, California, 1998.

Domar, Alice and Henry Dreher. *Healing Mind. Healthy Woman.* Delta, Bantam, New York, 1996.

Fielding, Helen. *Bridget Jones's Diary.* Picador, London, 1996.

Ford, Gillian. *Listening to Your Hormones.* Prima, Rocklin, California, 1995.

Francis-Cheung, Theresa. *Help Yourself Cope with the Biological Clock: How to Make the Right Decisions About Motherhood.* Hodder and Stoughton, London, 2001.

——. *Androgen Disorders in Women: The Most Neglected Hormone Problem.* Hunter House, California, 1999.

——. *Pregnancy Weight Management.* Adams Media Corporation, Holbrook, Massachusettes 2000.

Friedan, Betty. *The Fountain of Age.* Simon and Schuster, New York, 1993.

Friedman, S. Ann. *Work Matters: Women Talk About Their Jobs and Their Lives.* Viking, New York, 1996.

Gittleman, Ann Louise. *Before the Change: Taking Charge of Your Perimenopause.* HarperSanFrancisco, San Francisco, 1998.

Greer, Germain. *The Whole Woman.* Transworld, Doubleday, London, 1999.

Hayflick, Leonard. *How and Why We Age.* Ballantine Books, New York, 1996.

Heyn, D. *Marriage Shock: The Transformation of Women into Wives.* Delta, New York, 1997.

Hodgson, Harriet. *Smart Aging: Taking Charge of Your Physical and Emotional Health.* John Wiley and Sons, New York, 1999.

Horne, James. *Why We Sleep.* Oxford University Press, Oxford, 1989.

Hutchinson, Germaine. *Transforming Body Image.* Crossing Press, Watsonville, California, 1998.

Hutton, Deborah. *Vogue: Beauty for Life.* Crown, Random, New York, 1994.

Jansen, Robert. *Overcoming Infertility: A Compassionate Resource for Getting Pregnant.* W. H. Freeman, New York, 1997.

Jong, Erika. *Fear of Flying*. Holt, Rinchart and Winston, New York, 1973.

Josselson, R. *Revising Herself: The Story of Women's Identity from College to Midlife*. OUP, New York, 1996.

Jovanovic, Lois, M.D. and Genell J. Subak-Sharpe, M.S. *Hormones: The Woman's Answerbook*. Ballantine, New York, 1992.

Kaye, Edita. *Fountain of Youth: The Anti-Aging Weight-Loss Program*. Time Warner, New York, 1998.

Knight, Lindsay. *Why Feeling Bad Is Good*. Hodder and Stoughton, London, 1996.

Lansey, Bruce. *Age Happens: The Best Quotes and Cartoons about Getting Older*. Meadowbrook, Simon and Schuster, New York, 1997.

Levine, Barbara. *Your Body Believes Every Word You Say*. Aslan Publishing, Boulder Creek, California, 1991.

Levinson, Daniel. *The Seasons of a Woman's Life: A Fascinating Exploration of the Events, Thoughts and Life Experiences That All Women Share*. Ballantine, New York, 1996.

McKenna, Elizabeth Perle. *When Work Doesn't Work Anymore: Women, Work and Identity*. Simon and Schuster, London, 1997.

Monahan, William. *Eat for Health*. Kramer, Tiburon, California, 1989.

Nelson, Miriam. *Strong Women Stay Slim*. Bantam Doubleday, New York, 1999.

Northrup, Christiane, M.D. *Women's Bodies, Women's Wisdom: Creating Physical and Emotional Health and Healing*. Bantam, New York, 1995.

Ornish, Dean. *Eat More, Weigh Less*. Harper Collins, New York, 1993.

——. *Love and Survival: The Scientific Basis for the Healing Power of Intimacy*. Harper Collins, New York, 1998.

Pert, Candice B., Ph.D. *Molecules of Emotion: Why You Feel the Way You Feel*. Scribner, New York, 1997.

Prevention Magazine Editors and Rodale Center for Woman's Health. *Age Erasers for Women: Actions You Can Take Right Now to Look Younger and Feel Great.* Rodale Press, Emmaus, Pennsylvania, 1994.

Redmond, Geoffrey. *The Good News About Women's Hormones.* Time Warner, New York, 1995.

Reilly, L. *Women Living Single: Thirty Women Share Their Stories of Navigating through a Married World.* Faber and Faber, Boston, 1996.

Rowe, John and Robert Kahn. *Successful Aging.* Dell, Random, New York, 1998.

Schaaf, Anne Wilson. *Women's Reality.* Harper and Row, New York, 1982.

Seaman, Barbara. *The Doctor's Case Against the Pill.* Hunter House, California, 1995.

Sears, Barry. *The Anti-Aging Zone.* Regan, Harper Collins, New York, 1999.

Sheehy, Gail. *New Passages: Mapping Your Life Across Time.* Harper Collins, London, 1997.

———. *Menopause: The Silent Passage.* Pocket Books, New York, 1993.

———. *Passages: Predictable Crises of Adult Life.* Bantam, New York, 1974.

Somer, Elizabeth. *Age-Proof Your Body: Your Complete Guide to Lifelong Vitality.* William Morrow and Company, New York, 1998.

Spillane, Mary, and Victoria McKee. *Ultra Age: Every Woman's Guide to Facing the Future.* Macmillan, London, 1999.

Stewart, Felicia; Felicia Guest; Gary Stewart; and Robert Hatcher. *Understanding Your Body: Every Woman's Guide to Gynecology and Health.* Bantam, New York, 1987.

Sundermeyer, Colleen A. *I Want My Body Back: Nutrition and Weight Loss for Mothers.* Perigee, New York, 1998.

Thomas, A. G. *The Women We Become: Myths, Folktales and Other Stories About Growing Older.* Prima, Rocklin, California, 1997.

Thurer, S. L. *The Myths of Motherhood: How the Culture Reinvents the Good Mother*. Houghton Mifflin, New York, 1994.

Tilsner, Julie. *29 and Counting: A Chick's Guide to Turning 30*. Contemporary Books, Chicago, 1998.

Viorst, J. *Necessary Losses: The Loves, Illusions, Dependence and Impossible Expectations That All of Us Have to Give Up in Order to Grow*. Fireside, New York, 1986.

Vliet, Elizabeth Lee. *Screaming to Be Heard: Hormonal Connections Women Suspect and Doctors Ignore*. M. Evans, New York, 1995.

Wolf, Naomi. *The Beauty Myth*. Random, New York, 1997.

———. *Promiscuities: The Secret Struggle for Womanhood*. Vintage, London, 1990.

About the Author

Theresa Francis-Cheung obtained her bachelor's degree from King's College, Cambridge University, and her master's degree from King's College, London University. She writes full time about women's health issues. Her books include: *Androgen Disorders in Women: The Most Neglected Female Hormone Problem* (1999), *Pregnancy Weight Management* (2000), *Cope with Your Biological Clock: How to Make the Right Decision about Motherhood* (2001), *Worry: The Root of All Evil* (2001), and *Men and Depression: Helping Him, Helping You* (2002). A professional dancer before retraining as a fitness teacher and health consultant, she has also taught in schools and colleges and worked in health publishing. She is married to her husband, Ray, and has a son, Robert.

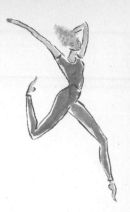

Index